DISCOVER POWERFUL T...
CAN GIVE YOU A GIFT OF H.......

• PRESSURE POINTS ON BOTH FEET TO LIFT YOUR
MOOD AND EASE DEPRESSION... AND HERBS
THAT HELP TOO

• WORK SPECIFIC AREAS OF THE FOOT TO SPEED
HEALING OF FRACTURES IN ANY PART
OF THE BODY

• OPEN LUNGS AND BRONCHI WITH THE TIP
AND EDGE OF YOUR THUMBS ON IMPORTANT
PRESSURE POINTS FOR BRONCHITIS

• FAST, EFFECTIVE RELIEF OF BACK PAIN FROM
REFLEXOLOGY... AND TAI CHI EXERCISES
FOR PREVENTION

• ALLEVIATE FATIGUE BY STIMULATING
EVERY MAJOR ORGAN

• PROMOTE A GLOWING, YOUTHFUL COMPLEXION
AND HELP TREAT ACNE AND OTHER
SKIN DISORDERS

THE HANDS-ON WAY TO HEALING...

THE PRESSURE POINT PLAN

THE PRESSURE POINT PLAN FOR NATURAL HEALTH

JUDITH BERGER
and
JUDITH SACHS

ibooks

DISTRIBUTED BY PUBLISHERS GROUP WEST

Distributed by Publishers Group West
1700 Fourth Street, Berkeley, CA 94710
www.pgw.com

An ibooks, inc. Book

ibooks, inc.
24 West 25th Street
New York, NY 10010

ISBN 1-59687-158-X
First ibooks, inc. printing November 2005

10 9 8 7 6 5 4 3 2 1

Printed in the U.S.A.

CONTENTS

located and give you a step-by-step program for your reflexology treatment.

INTRODUCTION

by Judith Berger

As more of us decide to take responsibility for our personal well-being, alternative and complementary medicine becomes more appealing. We have so many healing options that can change the nature of the way we feel, hour to hour, day to day, and year to year. Reflexology is an extraordinary natural therapy that can make daily life a lot more pleasant, can keep us in good health, and can nip incipient illnesses in the bud. If we are seriously ill, reflexology can serve as an excellent companion to conventional medical treatment.

When I began practicing reflexology in 1989, no one I knew had ever heard of it, and the people I talked to about it were usually dubious or amused—frequently both. My husband was skeptical when I was first learning until I started using him as a guinea pig. He quickly found that backaches, sinus congestion, and other day-to-day aches and pains responded very quickly to one of my sessions. As I offered my services around, a few friends took me up on it, not expecting very much besides relaxation and a nice foot massage. As time went on, however, clients began to see the results of treatment and came back for more . . . and they told *their* friends.

Often one individual would be in extreme discomfort from a condition that had not responded to conventional medical care, and I would be called in. Most of the time I would be able to effect a positive change in the condition of my client within two or three sessions, sometimes on the very first visit.

Reflexology, though not yet a mainstream treatment, has joined the ranks of other alternative and complementary therapies that take care not just of the problem in question but of the whole person. The way it works is very basic. Reflexology opens energy channels, breaks down blockages, and removes toxic calcium deposits from the body. It also pinpoints organs that are connected to the original problem organ through an intricate network of cells and tissues. When you work on the immune system as well as the sore shoulder, the whole body gets better faster. When you work on the whole spine as well as the head and neck to treat a migraine headache, you are looking at the bigger picture.

Although science has not yet been able to tell us how it works, reflexology is nearly always successful in its healing approach. It can also work beautifully in concert with conventional medical treatment to make the body respond more efficiently to medication and surgery. When you start to use this therapy, you'll prove it for yourself. This will allow you to benefit from many opportunities for growth that might otherwise have passed you by, making life much more interesting in the process.

Another asset of reflexology is its accessibility. The

feet are always there, always ready to be treated. Using reflexology will teach you how valuable these work-horses of the body really are; they are so well designed and well suited to their jobs. Those delicate adjustments of balance, the shifting of weight and propulsion through space: They do it all, something for which we should be very grateful.

One of the wonderful things about reflexology is its simplicity. Anyone can do it for him- or herself and for others, with some basic instruction and a little practice. With this book I hope to make a very valuable healing technique accessible to a great many people.

Judith Sachs and I have tried to make *Reflexology: The A–Z Guide to Healing with Pressure Points* the most concise and comprehensive foot reflexology guide available. With specific explanations of the philosophy and techniques of this therapy and descriptions of most common ailments and their treatment—each entry in alphabetical order with its own clear illustration—you have an excellent guide to help you on your journey to better personal health.

Rising health care costs have made a lot of people think twice before running to the doctor to correct minor imbalances in their daily health. The more we can do ourselves, the more we take charge of our own wellness, the better off we are. Reflexology is a holistic tool that belongs in the lexicon of natural treatments that will improve our general well-being today and for years to come.

CHAPTER ONE

What Is Reflexology?

Reflexology is the art of pressing points on the foot to balance energy and enhance healing elsewhere in the body. It is based on the idea that disease occurs when the body or any of its organs are overly stressed or out of balance. Reflexology causes a relaxation response throughout the many body systems that brings circulation back to normal and allows oxygen and nutrients to flow to the cells. As equilibrium is restored, healing can take place.

How Reflexology Works

Reflexes are involuntary responses to a stimulus carried by the nerves from one location to the next. What you do when you press, knead, and glide along various points is trigger neural connections from the foot up to the various organs. In so doing, you can balance the whole body, improve circulation, release blockages that may cause disease, and remove impurities and toxins.

And as you touch and move a point on the foot, you are able to send energy from this point throughout all the corresponding organs of the body.

Understanding the concept of energy is essential to understanding how reflexology works. In Eastern medicine the body is considered a channel for energy, a word that implies "life force" as well as "aliveness" or "alertness." In Chinese the word is qi (or chi), in Japanese it's ki, but they mean the same thing. This powerful guiding force, when blocked or stagnant, can interfere with good health throughout the body. By allowing energy to flow freely, the body can begin to heal itself.

In Chinese medicine the qi travels through blood and oxygen along pathways known as meridians, almost like underground tunnels that snake throughout the various organs and body systems. Although reflexology does not work on the meridian theory, a similar type of flow occurs in this therapy. Pressing on foot reflexes, we free up blocked energy, and this can alleviate a symptom and at the same time boost immune function so that the symptom won't recur.

If you look at a river running freely, you see a system functioning at its peak performance level. Fish swim; pollutants travel downstream; the leaves and mosses are washed by the movement of the water. But if a tree falls into the river, the branches form a dam, and regular activity grinds to a halt. Now the fish can't get their proper nourishment, toxins pool, and vegetation dries out.

In the same way the theory of reflexology holds that when energy is blocked in the body, it causes illness. If we hold so much tension in our shoulders that we restrict circulation, or we worry so much that our adrenal glands put out an excess of stress hormones, our energy becomes stagnant. In order to get it moving again, we have to break up the "dam" and wash away the accumulated toxins. Reflexology can help accomplish this goal.

The theory of pressure point healing is certainly not new. Many Native American Indian tribes have used reflex points to treat diseases of the internal organs for centuries. Chinese acupuncture and Japanese shiatsu manipulate the energy in various internal organs and tissues with needles and finger pressure. In the art of reflexology, the points used are those on the bottom, top, and sides of the foot. Specific reflex points on the foot correspond to specific areas throughout the body. According to the theory of reflexology, the physical action of working on these points in the feet breaks up the toxins that impede the flow of blood, oxygen, and energy.

When you learn the powerful techniques of reflexology, you can give yourself a gift every day, working your whole foot for general wellness and the specific points that relate to any physical problems you may be having. You can also give reflexology treatments to those you love and spread the wealth a little farther.

THE HEALTH BENEFITS OF REFLEXOLOGY

Here are just a few beneficial results of a reflexology session:

- By working points in the chest area, you can get steadier, more comfortable breathing and a calmer, less rapid heartbeat.
- By working the thymus gland at the base of the sternum, you can stimulate the immune system to produce antibodies to disease.
- By stimulating the pituitary gland in the brain, you can

rebalance the entire endocrine system and, by exten-
sion, all the hormones in the body.
- By stimulating the spleen, you can activate immune
responses to help fight infection.
- When you work the liver and kidneys, you can get rid
of toxins and stimulate waste elimination.

Another wonderful benefit of reflexology is immediate relief of a temporary problem. For example, if
you've just indulged in a rich, cholesterol-laden meal,
you can work on the liver points (since the liver is the
major site of cholesterol production and synthesis in the
body), and this will help alleviate stress on the organ as
you digest; if you've been up all night studying or have
been staring at the road throughout a six-hour car drive,
you can work on the eye points to take away tension;
and even right after a heart attack, while you're lying in
a hospital bed receiving drugs and other medical care,
you can ask a friend to work on the heart zone so that
the medication can work with greater speed and effec-
tiveness.

How Energy Blockages Cause Disease

Before we stood on two feet, we were more balanced
creatures. We used all our limbs to move around, to
grasp food and tools, to shelter ourselves from the elements and from natural enemies. But when we became
bipeds and stood erect, gravity began to influence our
health. Inorganic waste matter—uric acid that builds up
in the kidneys; lymph fluid that collects when lymph
glands in the groin, armpit, or neck are inflamed; calcium deposits that leach into the bloodstream instead of
staying in the bone—tends to be pulled downward by
gravity and builds up in the feet. These deposits can
impinge on muscles and nerves and in turn can create

new problems in the body. But working on the feet breaks up these deposits so that energy can flow.

Lymph fluid is transported mechanically as our muscles move and during respiration. If we hold a great deal of tension in one zone, lymph fluid can pool in corresponding areas of the feet.

Many of my clients tell me that they can feel an area in the foot that "crunches" when I show them how to work on it. These classic crunchy places indicate deposits or calcifications that have formed in the feet as the result of poor circulation and blocked energy. After the clients have worked the particular points for a few sessions, however, this "crunchy" sensation vanishes. That's the sign that the body is healing itself.

A CASE IN POINT

When I first began to practice reflexology, I was convinced that I would be able to alleviate tension and pain in clients with average complaints—an aching knee, chronic headaches, menstrual problems—but I was slightly apprehensive when a friend recommended that I treat Alva, a sixty-three-year-old woman with emphysema who had been housebound for a couple of months.

When I started treating Alva, it was with the hope that I would at least be able to reduce some of her stress and help her relax. Since emphysema, a serious lung disease, prevents the sufferer from getting enough oxygen, I thought that at the very least I would be able to open some energy channels and make her breathing a little easier.

Her feet were cold when I started working on them, and just the act of warming them with my hands seemed to make her feel better. I started with a general treatment of the entire foot and then worked the affected reflexes—the lungs and bronchi, the throat, the upper lymphatics, the diaphragm, the sternum, the solar plexus (to reduce tension), and the ileocecal valve (to alleviate excess mucus). Then I went on to work the causal reflex zones: the neck, the shoulder girdle, the digestive system (including the small intestine), the endocrine system (particularly the adrenal glands), and the spleen, heart, and spine.

I went to see Alva once a week for two years, and although progress was slow, she invariably got a great deal of relief from the sessions. Her doctors were constantly amazed at the difference in her whole attitude over time; the benefits she got from her treatments not only alleviated her symptoms, but definitely affected her general health and well-being.

Get to Stress Before It Gets to You

One of Alva's chief problems was that she lived with the stress of being chronically ill. When you feel you can't cope—with your sickness, your job, your relationship—you begin to build up toxins that the body can't release.

Stress is everywhere, and when it hits, the most common reaction is to take it inside and make it part of you. If you're stopped by a policeman for speeding, you get two varieties of stress at once: You get an expensive ticket, and at the same time you start the process of giving yourself a "guilt" ulcer for reckless driving. As soon as you're stressed, you have an immediate fight-or-flight reaction; you must instantly do something to preserve yourself. So your brain tells your adrenal glands to begin pouring out stress hormones (adrenaline, noradrenaline, and cortisol), your heart rate and blood pressure skyrocket, your breathing becomes shallow, your muscles tense, and the blood vessels on the surface of your skin contract.

Over time repeated stress reactions deplete vitamins

and minerals (especially vitamin C and the B vitamins) from the body. You produce more of the "bad" (LDL) cholesterol that adheres to your arteries and compromises your heart, and your immune system is weakened. If your life is incredibly stressful, your entire system may become unbalanced, you're drained of energy, and various dysfunctions or conditions can develop.

The most immediate way to lower this high pitch of the nervous system is to relax. A body conditioned to let go can roll with the punches and take life a little easier.

WELL-BEING AND REFLEXOLOGY

Reflexology is a wonderful tool for long-term stress relief. Since stress builds up a lot of calcium and lymph deposits in the feet, reflexology is also helpful in a purely mechanical way: A treatment can break up and reduce these deposits, thus alleviating problems elsewhere in the body. Because of the alternating pressure used on all different parts of the feet during a treatment, the corresponding areas throughout the body can be retuned and restored to normal functioning. When a specific foot point is manipulated, this relaxes tension at the site, lets the blood supply flow unimpeded, and makes nerve connections more accessible. Oxygen and nutrients can go where they're supposed to. And energy can flow from point to point, making you feel whole again.

Because we are not simply a collection of limbs and organs but rather one organism with its own method of checks and balances, we can channel healing properties throughout the system if we know how. It's important to realize that manipulating points on the foot can strengthen your immune system. This in turn will prevent you from contracting illnesses or may hasten your recovery if you are sick.

If you have a diagnosed illness or if you are having persistent symptoms that are interfering with your daily life, *you must be under the care of a medical practitioner.* Most Western-trained physicians aren't familiar with reflexology, so it may be helpful for you to sit down with your physician and explain how you'd like to use this therapeutic technique as a complement to traditional allopathic (Western) medicine. Most doctors will not object to your decision to use reflexology.

Even if you have a heart condition, you could tell your physician that you will be taking your daily medication and at the same time will be working the heart reflex point and other related points on your foot to improve circulation and enhance your body's healing abilities. If you have asthma, you can still use your inhaler while you work on your lung reflexes and other related points for better respiration. If you've just had an operation, you could explain to your surgeon that you will be helping your body make a faster and less painful recovery by pressing on reflex points related to your condition.

The reason that reflexology works so well as an adjunct to conventional medicine is that it is able to restore internal equilibrium and allow the body to begin the process of healing itself. It is both a preventive tool and a means of rebalancing circulation and energy, and it can release blockages in the body that may have helped cause illness or dysfunction. It can also help heal conditions that you've brought on yourself.

REFLEXOLOGY IS NOT MASSAGE

It should be pointed out that reflexology is quite different from massage, which works directly on a portion of the body to relax it and allow energy to flow more freely through the muscles and ligaments. Massage feels good because it involves personal touch, so a foot massage is certainly a sensual, enjoyable experience, but it cannot be classified as a reflexology session.

When you know your points and what organs, glands, and tissues they relate to, you are investing in a much more powerful system of healing. In reflexology you are accessing internal organs via external stimulation.

Whole body massage is a wonderful adjunct to foot reflexology, and doing some manipulative work with the area of the body you're trying to heal can enhance the effect of a reflexology treatment. As a matter of fact, the woman who pioneered reflexology as we know it today was a massage therapist. So the two can work hand in hand to attack the problem from different perspectives and give the body two intertwining avenues of healing.

THE HISTORY OF FOOT REFLEXOLOGY

Reflexology is a relatively new art in the healing lexicon. It was first developed by Dr. William Fitzgerald in the early 1900s. He saw that direct pressure on certain areas in the body could anesthetize others. Fitzgerald formulated a picture of the body as an entity divided into ten vertical zones that go through all organs and tissues (see the Zones of the Body, p. 12). As he saw it, a problem in one area of a zone could be helped by stimulating another place in the same zone.

A colleague of Fitzgerald's, Dr. Edwin Bowers, took reflexology one step farther. He saw that if you pressed on a certain point in a patient's hand at the same time that you stuck a pin in his face, he would feel no pain.

Then, in the early 1930s, a massage therapist named Eunice Ingham advanced reflexology to the art it is today. Using Fitzgerald's zone theory, she created a map of the body that corresponded to various areas on the feet. (She believed that we could derive more benefit from working on the feet than on the hands because the feet were protected by shoes most of the time and were therefore highly sensitive when stimulated.)

By experimenting, she figured out that alternating pressure on the designated points would work better than direct pressure, and she was astonished and delighted to find that her treatments offered much more than simple pain relief. Her patients began to describe a reduction or an elimination of symptoms, even of illnesses that had plagued them for years.

ZONE THEORY IN THE PRACTICE OF REFLEXOLOGY

Reflexology holds that energy flows through the body along ten designated pathways, known as zones. When Dr. Fitzgerald first saw the promise of pressing points in one place to alleviate pain in another place, he needed guidelines that would allow him to find his way from point to point. So he divided the standing human figure from the tips of the toes to the top of the head and also through the body three-dimensionally. (This is similar to the meridian theory in Chinese medicine, which designates fourteen pathways along which energy is directed throughout the body.) The ten reflexology zones are mirrored on the bottom of the foot, so that every organ and gland can be located on the foot as it is on the body.

Each finger and its corresponding toe as well as everything along that dividing line are in the same zone. Zone 1 runs along the center line of the body and moves outward to Zone 5 on the sides of the body. Zone 1 is also the area around the big toe and the thumb, fanning out to Zone 5 at the pinkie and little toe. The same reflex point from one zone can be found on the front and back of the body and on the top and bottom of the foot.

The right foot takes in all the organs on the right half of the body; the left foot encompasses the left half.

The entire body is represented on the bottom of the foot, and this is why it's important to work the whole foot, not just the particular reflex points that relate to the affected organ, when you do your reflexology treatment.

In addition to the ten vertical zones, there are three transverse zones that divide the internal organs of the body crosswise. The first goes from the top of the head down to the upper part of the shoulders and includes structures of the head and neck; the second goes down to the waist and takes in the structures of the thorax and upper abdomen; and the third ends at the bottom of the pelvic floor and includes organs of the lower abdomen and pelvis. (The legs and feet are not represented in the transverse zones because they contain no functional organs.)

If you're tense or congested anywhere on a zone, that tension or congestion affects the whole zone. This is similar to having a blockage in an artery that will affect blood flow throughout the body. At the same time direct pressure on any part of a zone affects the whole zone; this is why you can work on the feet and get relief in the head.

IS REFLEXOLOGY FOR EVERYBODY?

Reflexology is a wonderful adjunct tool for healing and can serve a multitude of purposes. It can be used on

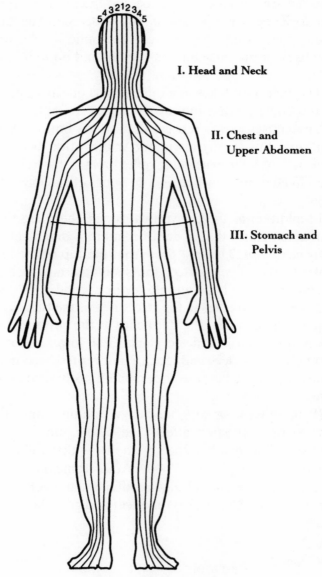

5 4 3 2 1 2 3 4 5

I. Head and Neck

II. Chest and
Upper Abdomen

III. Stomach and
Pelvis

The Zones of the Body

healthy people for toning and support to various organ systems; it can be used for those who've recently had traumatic injuries or those with long-term chronic illnesses. It's good for people of any age, including small children and the elderly.

There are a few cautions you should heed, however. During pregnancy it is vital that you avoid certain reflex points. The point on the inside of the heel right below the anklebone must *never* be used at this time, because it might stimulate contractions and begin a premature labor. However, this same point can be extremely useful to a nonpregnant woman who suffers from PMS or heavy cramps to make monthly periods easier.

If you have an extremely painful injury—for example, a broken ankle or a dislocated shoulder—you may want to go very gently on the foot that corresponds to that side of the body and work more firmly on the opposite foot.

If you fall and hurt your hip, and the next day your shoulder hurts as well, it's not surprising. The reason is that certain reflex points cover different locations in the same zone. The hip and shoulder points are identical, as are the elbow and knee and wrist and ankle. If you are working your hip and notice some sensitivity in your shoulder, it's because the entire zone is out of balance.

HOW TO USE THIS BOOK

Reflexology: The A–Z Guide to Healing with Pressure Points is a practical, hands-on primer of this healing art. This first chapter serves as an introduction to the theory of reflexology. And then we get right down to nuts-and-bolts information you need to practice this therapy on yourself or to teach a friend or relative to do it for you.

Chapter 2 will offer a clear picture of the European style of manipulating the feet with your hands. We'll describe the exact method of gliding and pressing on a lubricated foot with your thumbs and fingers. We'll show you how to take a break from the intense pressure of a reflexology session by relaxing and soothing the foot with twisting, rotating, and rocking motions.

Chapter 3 is a whole foot and whole body workout. In order to get the true benefits of reflexology, you want to begin each time with a head-to-toe reflexology session before treating a specific symptom or condition. We'll make clear which referral glands or organs might be treated in addition to the affected part. In other words, to take care of an earache, you work not only the ear point but also the adrenals to assist in reducing inflammation.

The main portion of the book, the A–Z guide, is an alphabetical listing of common diseases and conditions. In every instance we'll show you a picture of the foot with the location of the specific reflexes drawn in. These areas follow the general reflexology chart on pages 30–31. You will note that the foot on those pages is divided into shapes that are either clear, shaded, or black, so that you can distinguish one from the other when they're all together. In the A–Z guide, those shapes are printed separately to indicate areas you should manipulate for your particular problem. The lightness or darkness of color does not in any way mean that you should work them more gently or firmly—they are colored purely to differentiate them from one another.

Then we will give a description of the problem and its possible symptoms and explain how to work the whole body first before going on to the specific affected areas as well as to referred glands or organs. We'll tell you the particular pressing technique or manipulation to use.

REFLEXOLOGY FOR BETTER HOLISTIC HEALTH

The common wisdom for a well-rounded program of preventive health care is to eat right, exercise daily, get enough sleep, clean up your habits (eliminating cigarettes and recreational drugs), and see your doctor for regular checkups.

Now, in addition, you have another healing therapy literally at your fingertips. As you learn to use reflexology to alleviate tension and break up blockages, you will soon feel renewed energy coursing through you. Using the reflex points to fine-tune your sense of physical well-being, you can turn stress into relaxation and pain into wellness. As your reflexology practice grows stronger, you will find balance in mind, body, and spirit.

The art and practice of reflexology can open a door that may lead to greater personal comfort and increasingly better natural health.

∗

CHAPTER TWO

How to Work the Feet

The actual physical work of reflexology isn't hard, but it must be precise if you are to get the greatest possible benefit. Naturally, when you're working on yourself, you don't have the leverage you'd have when working on a partner, so it's a good idea to practice on a friend every once in a while. Also, this way you'll have feedback from someone else; what feels right to you doesn't necessarily do the trick for another person.

It's worth mentioning that reflexology should feel good, even when you come up against a "crunchy" area that indicates there's some disruption in the body's balance or harmony. For this reason, cut your nails short before you treat yourself or anyone else, and keep them that way. When an area hurts, the affected organ really needs work, so treat yourself gently!

Some Rules of "Thumb"

The basics can be stated very simply. Just keep in mind that there are exceptions to every rule. But for the most part:

- One hand holds the foot steady; the other works the reflex points.
- The thumb does all the work (with a little help from the index finger). Sometimes you'll use both thumbs, steadying the foot with the palm and other fingers of both hands. For this reason, it's important to practice your techniques with both hands; eventually you'll develop even strength and flexibility on the right and left sides.
- The types of movement you'll use are direct pressure (pressing straight down with your thumb), circular pressure (moving the thumb in a small circle over the reflex point), direct circular pressure (pressing down as you move your thumb in a circle), and gliding (pushing the thumb from one area to the next as you apply pressure).

Gripping, Pulling, and Pressing

Everyone knows how to hold an object: You just use your opposable thumb and grasp with your fingers. It's so routine you no longer think about the mechanics of using the hands and fingers as tools with which to work.

But to be a really expert reflexologist, it's best to start with a beginner's mind, as though you really had no idea how to grip, pull, or press.

Open your hand, then close the fingers into the palm with the knuckles curled in. Use first a gentle grip, then a stronger one. Now try it on the top of your foot. Lay the toes in your palm, and close the fingers over them.

Place the thumb on the bottom, and get a really good purchase on the arch. Try your grip on the side of the foot, then on the heel. Play around with your fingers on your toes until you feel confident.

Now it's time to experiment with a pulling action. Grip the top of the foot with flattened fingers, and place the thumb under the arch of the foot. Grip tightly, putting more pressure first on the thumb, then on the fingers. Now let your shoulder and elbow relax, and pull the foot away from the lower leg. At the same time concentrate on pulling your hand away from your arm. If you use your back muscles for pulling, your arm won't get as tired. Always keep your shoulder and elbow down while you're working.

Pressing is the most important movement in reflexology. Take a thick sponge, and practice pressing your thumb down into it, letting up the pressure just a little, then applying more pressure. Pay attention to the way it gives and springs back; your foot will do the same. When you're working on reflex points, you never want to apply constant pressure over a long time; this can deaden the area and slow down circulation and may adversely affect the whole zone. Instead allow a lot of play in your thumb as you press in and out.

Always start the pressing gently and gradually, and apply more strength as you go. Then back out of the pressure slowly; with no unexpected or jarring moves, you will move energy more efficiently.

How to Use Your Hands and Fingers

You'll find a variety of descriptions below for what to do and how to move. Let's be specific about the vocabulary so that you learn each movement correctly:

"Work" means to perform the required movements and apply the appropriate pressure to the area.

"Glide" means to push the thumb—sometimes heavily and sometimes lightly—across the reflex.

"Apply direct pressure" means to push straight down, as though you had a plumb line between your thumb and the reflex point. It's important to refer to your diagram of the foot at first (see pp. 30–31) so that you'll hit just the right spot.

"Apply gradual pressure" means to start by touching the reflex and then slowly give a little more and a little more until you are working deeply. You can apply gradual pressure directly or in a circular pattern.

"Apply circular pressure" means to give equal pressure as your thumb tip or edge circles in a clockwise or counterclockwise direction. Don't let up as you come around the circle; keep the pressure steady.

"Apply gradual circular pressure" means to start lightly on the surface of the skin as your thumb tip or edge circles the reflex and then slowly to give more pressure as your circles deepen.

"Work with a circular motion" means that rather than zero in on the point, you are moving around it, your hand and thumb rotating as you work.

"Tip of thumb" is the very end, right under the most rounded part of the nail.

"Pad of thumb" is the fleshy part in the center of the thumb, where you can see the whorl of your thumbprint.

"Edge of thumb" is the side. If you are right-handed, you will usually use the outside (left) edge; if you are left-handed, you will usually use the outside (right) edge.

"End of thumb" includes the tip and also the next quarter inch or so before the pad.

"Necks of toes" are the long pieces between the fleshy pad of the ball of the foot and the toe points. The neck ends at the demarcation line before the rounded tops of the toes.

"Base of toes" is the area just below the necks, where the toes meet the foot.

European versus American Reflexology Techniques

This book is based on European reflexology, which primarily uses the thumbs to apply pressure on lubricated reflex points. A small amount of lotion (never oil) is used to get the foot ready for treatment, and because it's slightly moist, the thumbs glide nicely, and the practitioner has greater sensitivity to what's going on under the surface of the skin. You'll find, as you begin to use reflexology on a regular basis, that if you don't use lotion, the friction of rubbing and pressing the feet is uncomfortable. Your techniques may also take a lot of dead skin off the area; that isn't harmful, but it may leave you feeling sensitive and raw.

For this reason, always use a lubricant. There are many excellent lotions on the market that are pleasant to use. You can experiment with good-quality hand lotion from the supermarket or explore exotic herbal products from health food stores and body shops.

Lubrication is a detecting device that helps in your investigation of what's wrong in the body. It's possible to feel whether individual points arc denser than others—indicating long-term congestion or imbalance—if there is crystallization present and how much, and how these elements change over time, as the body begins to react favorably to treatment. As a matter of fact, changes in the way an affected reflex point feels can sometimes be detected within the course of one treatment.

If you don't use lotion, you're doing American-style reflexology. There is also a difference in technique: In this practice, you use thumb-walking and finger-walking as well as manipulations with knuckles, fists, and palms.

There are also a variety of twisting, turning, and grinding hand techniques to manipulate the feet.

The style of work described in this book is actually simpler, so that you can learn it quickly and use it efficiently.

How to Use Your Thumbs

To a reflexologist, the first joint of the thumb is the most important organ in the body. It is the workhorse of this therapy, and it must be strong and sensitive at the same time. You have to feel your way from reflex to reflex, organ to organ, you have to be aware of crunchy areas that signal distress in the body, and you have to be versatile in your ability to use all parts of the thumb: tip, edge, pad, end, and entire surface.

Your thumbs will eventually become very strong with practice, but as with any physical activity, you may get sore if you work too hard too soon. Start out with lighter pressure and shorter treatments to avoid straining your hands. Make sure you don't hyperextend your thumbs backward (this can happen easily if you're double-jointed, as I am). You will become more and more intuitive, using varying amounts of pressure, as your hands learn to sense the skin, the muscles, and the ligaments and bones as well as the imbalances and blockages you will encounter.

For practice in gliding your thumb, you may wish to use your other hand instead of your foot since it's easier to reach and it's bare most of the time so that you can practice anywhere when you have a few free minutes.

Take a little hand lotion, and apply it. Take off any excess with a tissue. Your hands should feel smooth but not too slippery. Start with the outside edge of your thumb, and place it on the fleshy pad of your opposite hand, just at the groove between the thumb and the fingers. First place the thumb gently on the point, then gradually press in. See how much pressure you can exert before slowly letting up on it. Rock the thumb slightly forward from the edge to the tip, on the inside edge of the nail. Repeat the exercise. Changing the grip of your hand, rock over to the inside edge of the thumb. Repeat the exercise.

Next you'll work on the pad. Usually the action with the pad of the thumb is circular, so practice applying gradual pressure to several points on your hand and moving the pad in circles, clockwise and then counterclockwise. Rock the pad forward so that you are on the end rather than the tip of your thumb. Work the end in circles, small ones and increasingly larger ones.

Now change hands, and repeat the exercises on the opposite side.

You may notice that your thumb feels stronger in one position than another and on your primary hand; that's just because you're not accustomed to using every portion of this digit. In time, with enough repetitions, you should develop two great strong thumbs.

When you feel comfortable working on your hand, switch to your feet. Once again, apply just enough lotion so that your feet feel smooth but not slippery. You'll find that there's a real difference between the planes and valleys of the foot, since it's a much more sensitive organ than the hand. When you're working on yourself, you'll have to change angles frequently to get the best purchase on the foot for the intensity and power you need as you press in.

You'll use thumb gliding when you're doing your whole foot/whole body workout before tending to whatever ailment you might have and also when you're concentrating on a large area like the spine or the intestines. In order to pinpoint a small area, stop your thumb gliding, and allow the thumb to hook into the point. Then pull back across this point with your thumb.

How to Use Your Fingers

Your four fingers will be holding the opposite side of the foot from your gliding thumb. Use the fingers to grip the toes, hold them back, and pull them forward. While you are gliding the thumb, your fingers can play back and forth as you raise and lower your wrist. Sinking your wrist increases pressure; raising your wrist decreases it.

You can also use the fingers for a broader expanse of pressure than you'll get with your thumb. For example, if you're working on the bronchial area, you can get your fingers in between the bones on the top of the foot. You put your thumb in the center of the sole of the foot (at the solar plexus reflex point) and tap your fingers one at a time (as though you were feeling impatient) in between the bones at the top of the foot. (Be sure not to put pressure directly on the bones, but rather, work in between them.)

Take a Break from Your Hard Work

It's important not to wear yourself out, particularly if you have an acute problem and are working reflex points that cause discomfort. The intensity of deep pressure should be alleviated every once in a while; too much constant pressure will deaden sensitivity to that area and may slow down circulation. Also, when you alternate intense and light touches, you can really feel the difference in both the reflex points and the affected body part. Of course, if you're working on a partner, he or she will appreciate taking a breather in the middle of a session. Good times to lessen your intensity are right after you've done your whole foot/whole body workout (see Chapter 3) and are about to go on to the specific condition or in between feet.

Let us say you have a headache and have just completed working on the reflexes for the whole body. Before you go on to the specific treatment for the headache, cradle each foot in your hands in turn, and rotate it. Then twist it side to side so that you feel a stretch between the arch and the toes and the heel.

Now make a fist, and press it into the arch of one foot. Use the knuckles to give a rolling massage. One by one, rotate them around, covering the entire sole and then the top of the foot. Repeat on the other foot.

Using your palms, flex the foot back and forth in your hand; now rotate it in a wide circle from the ankle, trying to hit every point as you move it clockwise, then counterclockwise. Finally, rock it slowly back and forth, as though it were a kitten or puppy lying along your hand and forearm. Repeat on the opposite side.

Grab the foot in the middle, pressing your thumb into the arch, and with the opposite hand, take the toes and flex them outward.

You will notice that you feel greatly relaxed after this break and ready to take on the deep work of the foot that lies ahead.

Always listen to your body. If you're going too quickly or slowly, make adjustments, and if you need time to let go of tension in the midst of a treatment, by all means, do so.

*

CHAPTER THREE

THE WHOLE FOOT/WHOLE BODY WORKOUT

A reflexology treatment involves priming, toning, and healing the entire body—head to toes, inside and outside. Just pressing on one point to take care of a particular problem isn't enough; your sessions should give every organ and tissue a workout. You can and should do treatments even when you feel fine in order to balance the body.

In this chapter you will get the basics of working the two feet to heal the whole body. In addition, you'll learn the location of all the points on both feet and the order of a reflexology treatment. All the maps of the feet—soles, tops, right and left ankles—are included here. You can refer back to this chapter as you need to in order to find particular landmarks on the feet and learn exactly how to manipulate them.

A Whole Body Workout for Better
General Health

Imagine that you can take a picture of yourself standing up that reveals everything inside you. Now reduce that photograph about 80 percent, and plaster it on the bottom of your foot. Just as the eyes are said to be the window to the soul, so the foot offers a vista of the whole human form. Your big toe matches your head; your eyes are just under the second and third toes; your ears are just under your fourth and fifth toes. The spine runs the length of the inner curve of the foot to the heel; the solar plexus is right in the center of the fleshy part of the ball, between the first and second toes, and the heart is found toward the outer curve of the top of the right foot, about half an inch under the fourth and fifth toes. There is a reflex point on the foot that corresponds to every organ, gland, and function in the body.

What the Feet Can Tell Us About the Body

When you're doing a treatment, pay attention to the texture, color, and odor of the feet. These external elements offer helpful clues to what's going on elsewhere in your system, both internally and externally.

If you look at the calluses on your soles, you'll note that some areas are thicker than others. It's possible that the reflex under this area is out of balance and the cause is elsewhere in the body. Calluses on the ball of the foot can affect your lungs. Corns or bunions on the toes can show up as neck or shoulder problems. Ingrown toenails put direct pressure on areas corresponding to the head, causing headaches or sinus problems.

Another important sign for you to learn to read is the discoloration you may see on your feet. If certain areas

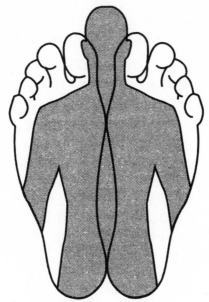

The Body in the Feet

are too red, this may mean that there is too much blood passing through the reflex. If there are white areas, your circulation may be poor. If you see purple patches, this means that there is some congestion.

The texture of the skin can also tell you a lot. Dry flaking on the bottom of your foot means that the corresponding area in the body lacks energy. Cracks in the skin or between the toes may mean the same thing.

You must also be aware of the temperature and odor of your feet. The more waste matter your body holds inside, the more your feet perspire and feel damp and clammy to the touch. A strong cheesy smell means heavy waste accumulation as well; a sharp acetone smell means some problem with the urinary tract.

You may notice, as you begin to treat yourself to re-flexology sessions, that your feet actually change in appearance, texture, and aroma. They should become more attractive and more comfortable as the corresponding problems in the body are attended to.

WARMING UP FOR A REFLEXOLOGY SESSION

A reflexology treatment should be a leisurely, enjoyable event, so start slowly, whether you are working on yourself or a partner. As with any exercise, you need to warm up before you get right into action.

Begin with some general relaxation techniques, such as a brief meditation or a visualization about the part of the body that concerns you and that you are going to help heal. Sit on the floor on a mat or carpet with your back well supported by cushions. Take some deep cleansing breaths, and stretch your feet out in space, circle them at the ankles, and flop them inward and outward, getting pigeon-toed and then into a dancer's first position with the heels together, toes facing away from each other.

When you are ready, bend your knees and bring your feet in toward your trunk. Grasp both feet in both hands, and massage them gently on the tops, bottoms, and sides. Then take one foot in both hands. Pull your top hand along the ankle, and pull the other on the tops of the toes in the opposite direction, as if you were trying to pull the foot off the leg. Extend your foot as far away from the body as it will go. Press your thumbs into the solar plexus points, and let your toes curl up and down around the pressure. Change feet, and repeat.

Draw your fingers down the length of the foot; run them along the tendons on the top of the foot, and then press the toes down, curling them under. Run them along the bottom of the foot from heel to toe, and press the toes back toward the body.

Interlace your fingers in your toes, and shake the toes back and forth, up and down.

Make a fist, press it into the soles of your feet, and rub the knuckles on each area: heel, pad, arch, ball.

Slap the foot gently with your hands to stimulate the skin.

End the warm-up by cupping each foot in both hands.

HOW TO LOCATE EACH ORGAN ON YOUR FOOT

Before you begin your treatment, you need to know how the body is divided on the bottom of the foot and where each organ sits in relation to the five zones. The following illustrations will show you exactly where each reflex lies. By using these maps, you can pinpoint the area you're concentrating on whether you're working your foot or someone else's. The more exact your location, the more benefit you receive.

The zones of the feet correspond to the zones of the body: Zone 1 runs from the big toes downward; Zone 5 runs from the fifth toe downward. (The big toes themselves are divided into five zones on each toe, 1 being on the interior edge, 5 being closest to the second toe.)

If at first you are confused about the location of a point, go back to your zone chart on page 12; you'll see, for example, that if you have an injured shoulder, it can be useful to work its neighbor in the zone, the hip. If you're working on the knee, you are affecting the elbow as well, because it's on the same reflex point.

The divisions of the feet and the corresponding body areas, in general terms, follow the expected order, from top to bottom:

Toes equal head and neck.

Balls of feet equal chest, lung, and shoulder.

Upper arch equals diaphragm to waist area.

Lower arch equals waist to pelvis.

Heel equals pelvic area to sciatic nerve.

Inside of foot equals spine.

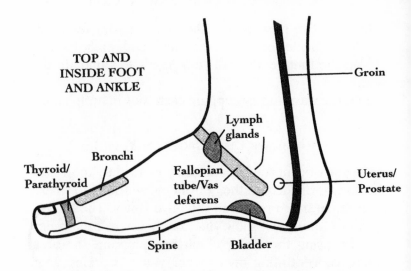

TOP AND INSIDE FOOT AND ANKLE

Groin

Lymph glands

Bronchi

Thyroid/ Parathyroid

Fallopian tube/Vas deferens

Uterus/ Prostate

Spine

Bladder

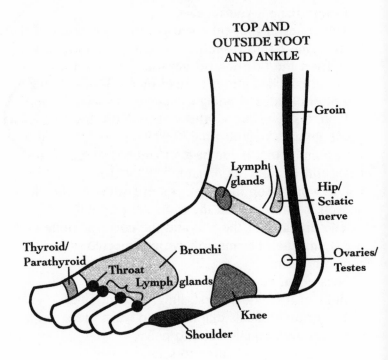

TOP AND OUTSIDE FOOT AND ANKLE

Groin

Lymph glands

Hip/ Sciatic nerve

Thyroid/ Parathyroid

Bronchi

Throat

Lymph glands

Ovaries/ Testes

Knee

Shoulder

SOLES OF FEET

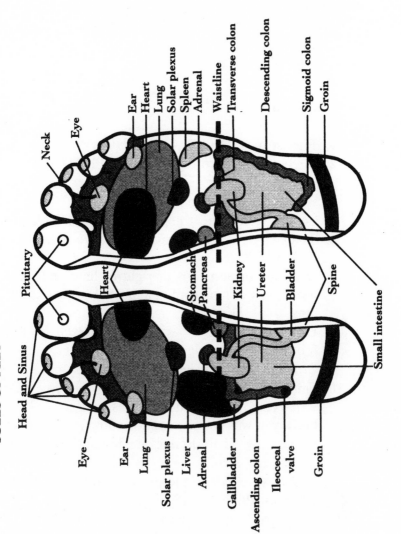

Outside of foot equals arm, shoulder, elbow, hip, leg, knee, and lower back.

Ankle area equals reproductive organs.

The Maps of the Feet

Soles of Both Feet

1. Tops of toes: HEAD AND SINUS
2. Circle in center of big toes, pad: PITUITARY
3. Second and third toes, pad: EYE
4. Fourth and fifth toes, pad: EAR
5. Center patch of feet above arch: CHEST/LUNG
6. Small circle directly in center above arch: SOLAR PLEXUS
7. Oval pad on left foot to right of lung and right foot to left of lung (but you must also work chest/lung area): HEART
8. Large patch directly across from spleen on left foot and liver on right foot: STOMACH
9. Circle in center of feet: KIDNEY
10. Small circle sitting on top of kidney: ADRENALS. (As you pull the toes back toward the body, you will notice a tendon running the length of the toes. The adrenals are inside this tendon, around the arch.)
11. Small half circle on the inside arch of feet below adrenals: PANCREAS
12. Large patch, centered but touching inner edge of feet: SMALL INTESTINE
13. Line dividing feet right through center of kidneys: WAISTLINE
14. Tube from inside edge of kidney to inside edge of feet an inch and a half down: URETER TUBE

15. Patch on inside edge of feet, two inches down from waistline: BLADDER
16. Tube on right foot to the left of the intestine, connecting to ascending colon and on left foot connecting to descending colon: TRANSVERSE COLON
17. Rest of heels: HELPER AREA TO LOWER BACK
18. Thin band running entire length of inside of feet: SPINE
19. Portion of spine from base of big toes to one inch below waistline: THORACIC SPINE
20. Portion of spine from an inch below waistline to top of heels: LUMBAR SPINE
21. Below lumbar: SACRUM
22. Below sacrum: COCCYX

Right Sole Only

1. Small bean shape on outer edge of liver: GALL-BLADDER
2. Beginning of ascending colon directly across from kidney near outside of right foot: ILEOCECAL VALVE
3. Tube on right foot connecting upward from ileocecal valve: ASCENDING COLON
4. Oval to right of solar plexus: LIVER

Left Sole Only

1. Band to left of solar plexus on left foot: SPLEEN
2. Tube on left foot directly across from ascending colon: DESCENDING COLON
3. Hook on left foot up from descending colon, ending in bladder: SIGMOID COLON

Top and Outside of Feet

1. Band across big toes under nail: THYROID/
   PARATHYROID
2. Circle below spaces between first and second
   toes: THROAT
3. Three circles below spaces between rest of toes:
   LYMPH GLANDS
4. Large patch in center of tops of feet: BRONCHI
5. Oval beneath pinkies: SHOULDER
6. Triangle above arches: KNEE
7. Band extending across tops of feet, bone to bone:
   FALLOPIAN TUBES/VAS DEFERENS
8. Oval in middle of band: LYMPH GLANDS
9. Boomerang shape next to anklebones: HIP/SCI-
   ATIC NERVE
10. Circle in the center of heels on outside: OVA-
    RIES/TESTES
11. Band running around side of ankles and under
    heels: GROIN

Top and Inside of Feet/Ankles

1. Band across big toes under nail: THYROID/
   PARATHYROID
2. Band below thyroid: BRONCHI
3. Long, thin band along bottoms of feet: SPINE
4. Band across tops of feet: FALLOPIAN TUBES/
   VAS DEFERENS
5. Oval in middle of band: LYMPH GLANDS
6. Half circle behind arches: BLADDER
7. Circle inside anklebones: UTERUS/PROSTATE
8. Band running around inside of ankles and under
   heels: GROIN

THE ORDER OF THE REFLEXOLOGY TREATMENT

Always do a whole foot/whole body workout before you treat your specific problem in order to balance all the body systems. Begin by working every reflex point in both feet, first the right foot, then the left, being sure that each point is equally stimulated. Next go on to work the reflexes for the particular ailment that concerns you. Now you can switch back and forth from foot to foot to encompass all the points for the organs where the left and right feet dovetail (as in the heart, the liver, or the colon). Remember to come back to the kidneys several times after working the other areas. The kidneys are crucial organs because they help process the toxins being released during a treatment and facilitate the proper functioning of the entire body.

In addition to working the points for the organ or area that needs attention, you should work the associated points that will reduce inflammation, stimulate immune system activity, increase energy in the body, and calm the anxious mind that might be worried about the illness.

The order of treatment isn't engraved in stone anywhere; if you vary what you do from time to time, it won't make any difference in terms of benefit. Just be sure you cover the whole body, stem to stern.

Right Foot

1. Work the sinus, head, and pituitary reflexes, beginning with the big toe and then working across the rest of the toes. Be sure to include the facial and jaw reflexes on top and around the nail of the big toe.

   Head/Sinus: Using thumb tip, first work tips of

toes using circular motion, then work all around the whole toe.

Pituitary: Apply direct pressure to reflex with thumb tip.

2. Move on to the neck and throat reflex. Then work the lymph glands at the base of the small toes.

Neck: Using thumb and index finger, manipulate "necks" of toes thoroughly.

Throat: Apply gradual direct pressure on reflex point on top of foot. (CAUTION: This can be painful.)

Lymph Glands: Work thumb gently back and forth across area, using tip and pad.

3. Work across the base of the toes, paying special attention to the eye and ear (including inner ear and eustachian tube) reflexes.

Eyes: Apply direct circular pressure with thumb tip.

Ears: Apply circular pressure with thumb tip.

4. Work the top of the foot, including the chest, lungs and bronchi, parathyroid/thyroid gland, fallopian tube, and hip/thigh/sciatic nerve.

Lungs: With the tip and edge of the thumb, work up and down and left to right.

Bronchi: With tip and edge of both thumbs, glide from the bases of the toes up toward the instep.

Thyroid/Parathyroid: Work "necks" of toes with thumb tip.

Fallopian Tube: Glide tip of thumb back and forth along area.

Hip/Thigh/Sciatic Nerve: Work thumb edge all around lower edge of outer anklebone.

5. Work your way across to the shoulder reflex at the "ball" of the little toe, then down the outside of the foot to work the knee/elbow.

Shoulder: Apply firm pressure to reflex with thumb tip.

Knee/Elbow: Work the end of the thumb all around the fifth metatarsal bone on the outside of the foot.

6. Work the diaphragm and solar plexus.

Diaphragm/Solar Plexus: With thumb tip, apply gradual pressure in the middle of the reflex and work out to the edges.

7. Work the stomach and pancreas.

Stomach: Apply gradual circular pressure with thumb tip and pad.

Pancreas: Apply direct circular pressure with thumb tip.

8. RIGHT FOOT ONLY: Work the liver and gallbladder.

Liver/Gallbladder: Apply direct pressure to gallbladder; then glide up and to left across liver.

9. Work the kidney, adrenal glands, bladder, and ureter.

Kidney: Apply direct pressure with thumb tip.

Adrenal Glands: Apply direct pressure with thumb tip.

Bladder: Apply circular pressure with thumb pad.

Ureter: Glide tip of thumb down ureter, from kidney to bladder.

10. RIGHT FOOT ONLY: Work the ileocecal valve, the ascending colon, and the transverse colon.

Ileocecal Valve (this valve is a sphincter muscle that works in only one direction. It connects the small intestine and the ascending colon and prevents food material from reentering the small intestine): Apply direct pressure with thumb tip.

Ascending Colon: Glide thumb tip from ileocecal valve up this reflex.

Transverse Colon: Glide thumb tip left to right across this reflex to the inside edge of the foot.

11. Work the intestines (gently if you have just eaten).

Small Intestine: Glide thumb back and forth and up and down through area.

12. Beginning at the base of the big toenail, work the entire spine from top to bottom.

Spine (Whole Back): Holding one foot with one hand, glide the other thumb tip from top to bottom of the reflex.

Upper Back (Cervical Spine): Glide thumb tip down the inside of the foot from the base of the big toe to the top of the ball of the foot.

Mid-back (Thoracic Spine): Glide thumb tip down inside of foot from base of the big toe to the bottom of the ball of the foot.

Lower Back (Lumbar Spine): Glide thumb tip down the inside of the foot from the base of the ball to the top of the heel.

Tailbone (Coccyx): Apply gentle circular pressure with thumb tip from the top of the heel to the bottom of the heel on the inside of the foot.

13. Work the pelvic area on the bottom of the heel; then move up toward the ankle, working the reproductive organs.

Groin: Apply firm thumb pad pressure throughout bottom of heel.

Ovaries: Apply gradual pressure with thumb tip and pad.

Uterus: Apply gradual circular pressure with thumb tip and pad.

Testes: Apply gradual circular pressure with thumb tip and pad.

Prostate Gland: Apply gradual circular pressure with thumb tip and pad.

Finish with a general relaxation for the entire foot similar to the warm-up. The sides of both ankles also contain several points that relax the whole body, so don't neglect them.

Left Foot

1. Work the sinus, head, pituitary.
2. Work the neck and lymph glands.
3. Work the eyes and ears.
4. Work the chest, fallopian tube, and hip.
5. Work the lung, bronchi, thyroid/parathyroid glands.
6. LEFT FOOT ONLY: Work the heart.
   Heart: Using thumb tip, work around reflex with circular motion.
7. Work the shoulder and the knee/elbow.
8. Work the diaphragm and solar plexus.
9. Work the stomach and pancreas.
10. LEFT FOOT ONLY: Work the spleen.
    Spleen: Apply gradual circular pressure with thumb tip and pad.
11. Work the kidney, adrenal gland, bladder, and ureter.
12. LEFT FOOT ONLY: From the inside edge of the foot, work across the transverse colon and down the descending colon to the sigmoid colon, ending at the rectum.
    Descending Colon: Glide thumb tip down this reflex.
    Sigmoid Colon: From descending colon, continue gliding thumb with a slight hook upward at the sigmoid colon.
13. Work the intestines.

14. Work the spine from top to bottom.
15. Work the pelvic area and reproductive organs.

Finish with a general relaxation for the entire foot similar to the warm-up. The sides of both ankles also contain several points that relax the whole body, so don't neglect them.

Next, move on to your healing session. Depending on your condition, select the sequence of reflexes (see A–Z listings) that will help remove blockages and toxins and get energy flowing to the affected area.

WORKING REFLEXES FOR HEALING

It's interesting to compare and contrast the way reflexology treats an ailment with the way conventional medicine treats it. If you suffer from heart disease and are under the care of a cardiologist, your first line of treatment will be medication—to lower blood pressure or cholesterol, to open blocked arteries, to eliminate excess water retention, or to adjust an irregular heartbeat. The second line of treatment will be a modified program of diet and exercise, again to lower blood pressure and cholesterol. The third line of treatment—if your doctor sees its worth—will be a structured program of stress reduction, because stress in and of itself can cause plaque to collect on arterial walls.

Reflexology works quite differently, but it's completely complementary to conventional medicine, so you can do both simultaneously. In a reflexology treatment the goal is to balance the energy around the heart reflex, but also around other reflexes that relate to the heart. The solar plexus and adrenals are important because they are involved in the stress/alarm reaction of the body. By balancing these points, you may be able to stave off the fight-or-flight response you get when you're stressed that triggers the production of damaging chemicals.

As you become more fluent with the reflex points, you'll discover how much better you feel when the entire foot is stimulated during the treatment. Then, and only then, can you move on to the specific disease or condition that requires your attention.

MOVING ON TO THE REFLEXES THAT YOU NEED MOST

Now you're ready to turn to the A–Z section and study the reflex points and types of manipulation that will help you heal many of your physical and emotional problems. Since reflexology works well in conjunction with other complementary therapies and treatments, we've included suggestions for preventive care and commonsense measures you can take as you make reflexology a part of your health care program.

The A–Z Guide

Acne

You wake up feeling fine and wander into the bathroom. You look in the mirror, and your spirits tumble. There is nothing as disheartening as seeing a pimple blossoming in a particularly obvious place. Acne—often a plague of adolescence—can strike at any age, and it seems to upset people in their fifties just as much as those in their teens. Why do we break out, and what can we do about it?

The skin is made up of many layers. The epidermis is on top, and beneath it is the dermis, which contains the shaft of a hair follicle. These follicles are lubricated by a sebaceous (oil-producing) gland that puts out a type of oil known as sebum. When too much sebum is produced, it can block up the top of the follicle, forming a blackhead and killing off the hair beneath. With an even greater increase of sebum production at this site, bacteria may gather in this area, breaking down the sebum into irritating fatty acids that attract pus cells. The follicle can then become inflamed and red, forming a pimple.

Another cause of skin disorders is an underdeveloped group of cells forming the lining of the hair follicle. These cells block pores so that they appear as blackheads or whiteheads.

Still another possible cause is hormonal. The male sex hormones (also produced in smaller amounts by women) known as androgens increase the size of oil glands and the quantity of oil produced. Women tend to break out prior to their periods, when they are producing more female sex hormones (estrogen and progesterone), which are not generally associated with oil gland regulation. But hormonal stimulation often causes a lot of emotional turmoil, and stress is sometimes associated with acne.

Finally, what you eat can sometimes make you break out, although scientific studies have proved that chocolate and other sweets are rarely the culprits. A great deal of fat in the diet on a regular basis, however, may encourage the development of pimples and blackheads. (Still, it's possible that people who have poor eating habits also have poor hygiene habits and just don't wash their faces as much as they should.)

But the underlying causes for the condition go beyond bacteria and blockages. Many people simply have a lot more oil in their skin than others. Sebum is more prevalent in some individuals. The abundance of this oil may or may not cause acne.

SYMPTOMS: Raised, red, often painful pustules on the face, chest, or back that may develop into angry-looking cysts. Small black, embedded areas (blackheads) or small hard white cysts (comedones) in the skin.

Areas to Treat/Types of Manipulation

Work both feet completely first. Then find the locations of reflexes that correspond to these organs, and work them in the following order (see Chapter 3 for guidance):

1. Kidneys: Apply direct pressure with thumb tip.
2. Thyroid: Work "necks" of toes with thumb tip.
3. Reproductive System: Apply gradual circular pressure with thumb tip and pad to ovaries and uterus (females) or prostate and testes (males).
4. Adrenals: Apply direct pressure with thumb tip.
5. Pituitary: Apply direct pressure with thumb tip.

Preventive Measures and Complementary Treatments

Reflexology works well in conjunction with other alternative therapies and commonsense measures. For example:

WASH YOUR FACE: Wash your face twice a day with warm water and mild soap, and wash your hair daily to keep down oil production. There are many medicated soaps and astringents on the market; you may have to experiment with several until you find one that works. Some dermatologists think that soap and water dry the face, and they are especially leery of abrasive creams or sponges that may remove natural skin oils.

USE BENZOYL PEROXIDE: Found in many over-the-counter preparations, this lotion, cream, or gel dries the skin, promotes peeling, and also keeps away the bacteria that create the damaging fatty acids in skin.

DON'T PICK OR SQUEEZE: Home treatments to remove blackheads or pimples can severely scar the skin. If you feel a need to get rid of the pustules on your face, have

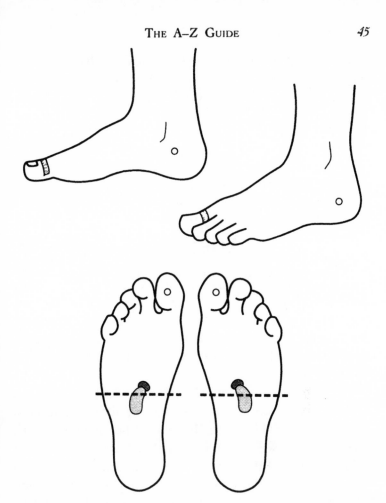

it done professionally by a trained cosmetician who does facials.

SEE THE SUN: If you are not using prescription medication, you may try sitting in the sun for half an hour every other day (wearing an SPF sunscreen of at least 8). The ultraviolet rays may help to dry the affected areas, but you must be exceptionally careful about taking precautions against sunburn. *If you are taking antibiotics, you must not get any sun exposure at all.*

You may wish to consult a physician who will prescribe antibiotics or tretinoin cream if neither reflexology nor any of the above complementary treatments clear up your acne. However, understand that it may take years to grow out of this condition whether or not you seek medical attention.

ADENOIDS

You can't breathe, and you know you look dumb with your mouth hanging open, but that's the only way you can get enough oxygen. Your partner tells you that your snoring every night is really annoying. When you speak, you're so nasal you sound as if you're whining all the time.

Adenoids are two small masses of lymphatic tissue that sit at the back of the nose directly above the tonsils. They're very valuable in that like other lymph glands, they produce white blood cells that help fight bacteria and viruses and therefore act as guardians of the respiratory system. These glands generally enlarge during childhood and start to shrink at about age fifteen.

If you have a throat infection or allergy, your tonsils and adenoids may also become enlarged as they become inflamed. Although they generally shrink after the infection has cleared, they sometimes remain enlarged, causing the classic nasal voice and contributing to postnasal drip. They may block not only the nasal passages but also the opening of the eustachian tubes, which may predispose a child to repeated ear infections and hearing loss.

SYMPTOMS: Adenoids may cause difficulty breathing,

openmouthed breathing, a nasal-sounding voice, snoring, pus drainage down the back of the throat, repeated inner ear infections, earaches, and hearing loss.

Areas to Treat/Types of Manipulation

Work both feet completely first. Then find the location of the throat reflex, and work it carefully (see Chapter 3 for guidance):

Throat: Apply gradual direct pressure on reflex point. (CAUTION: This can be painful.)

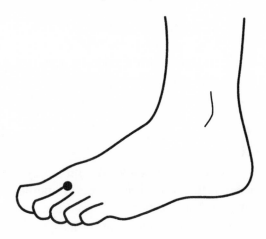

Preventive Measures and Complementary Treatments

Reflexology works well in conjunction with other alternative therapies and commonsense measures. For example:

BREATHE EASY TEA: Sit over a pot of chamomile tea with a towel over your head, and breathe in. Be sure to open your throat and allow the warmth to pervade your whole upper respiratory system.

TAKE A PREVENTIVE HERB: If you feel a cold coming on,

take half a dropperful of goldenseal and echinacea three times daily to strengthen the immune system.

If reflexology and the alternative therapies listed above have not provided relief, if you always have difficulty breathing or hearing, or if you have repeated ear infections, consult your physician, who may recommend a course of antibiotics or, for severe problems, surgery.

ALLERGIES

Is there a cat in the room? Suddenly you itch all over, and you feel a hive forming on your face. It's hard to breathe, and your eyes are watering so much you can't see three feet in front of you.

Allergies are acute immune system responses to a particular antigen, or foreign agent. When the body is sensitive to an element in the environment—a type of food, pollen, insect bites or stings, animal dander, certain medications, and hosts of other possible elements—it forms antibodies—specialized proteins—to fight the invasion. Antibodies then combine with the antigen so as to defuse its harmful properties and sometimes mark it in a certain way so that the body's macrophages, or scavenger cells, can more quickly recognize and destroy it.

There are four types of antigens: those you inhale (dust, pollen, dander, feathers), those you ingest (particularly chocolate, strawberries, milk, eggs, shellfish, peanuts, tomatoes, and citrus fruits), those that are injected (insect or jellyfish venom), and those you make physical contact with (poison ivy or oak, cosmetics, detergents, fabrics, or dyes).

Your first exposure to an allergen may cause an instant reaction, although this is not the common pattern. For most people it takes time to develop allergies, as the immune system girds itself for the next exposure by forming appropriate antibodies. The antibodies stimulate special cells to produce histamine, a chemical that dilates blood vessels and constricts smooth muscles in the respiratory system and digestive tract and also forms hives, which are raised, itchy red patches on the skin. You may tolerate a substance for years and then suddenly develop a sensitivity to it; conversely, you may be allergic to something and then one day find that you don't have any reaction to it at all. No one is really sure why this is true, although it's clear that certain individuals are much more prone to allergies than others.

There may be a psychogenic component to allergies; feeling a great deal of stress and fear around cats or bees, for example, could give you a more heightened sensitivity than feeling neutral about them.

SYMPTOMS: Watery eyes, runny nose, sneezing, itching locally or over entire body surface, inflamed skin, formation of hives, swollen mouth or throat. A serious and potentially life-threatening allergic reaction, known as anaphylactic shock, can constrict the airways so severely, swelling the throat, larynx, and bronchial tubes, that it becomes impossible to breathe.

AREAS TO TREAT/TYPES OF MANIPULATION

Work both feet completely first. Then find the locations of reflexes that correspond to these organs, and work them in the following order (see Chapter 3 for guidance):

1. Adrenals: Apply direct pressure with thumb tip.
2. Reproductive System: Apply gradual circular pres-

sure with thumb tip and pad to ovaries and uterus (females) or prostate and testes (males).

3. Pituitary: Apply direct pressure with thumb tip.
4. Bronchi: With the tip and edge of thumbs, glide from the base of the toes up toward the instep.
5. Lungs: With the tip and edge of thumb, work up and down and left to right.

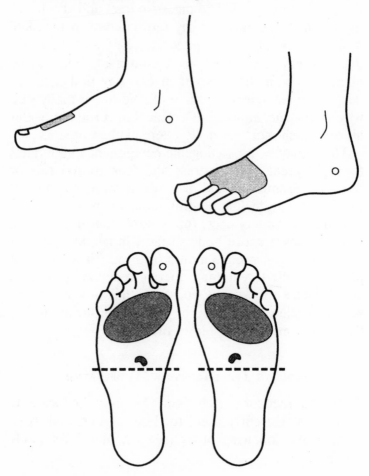

PREVENTIVE MEASURES AND COMPLEMENTARY TREATMENTS

Reflexology works well in conjunction with other alternative therapies and commonsense measures. For example:

BREATHE COOL, DRY, CLEAN AIR: The more you can stay in air-conditioning, the better. You may wish to buy a dehumidifier for your bedroom and an industrial-quality air cleaner for your central heating and cooling unit.

PET ISOLATION: If you react badly to pets, you shouldn't have any. But if you adore them, or your kids insist, be sure you assign someone grooming chores. Brushing and combing (outside, if possible) will keep the dander down. Also, give your animals one room of their own and make the others off-limits.

WASH YOUR BEDDING: Mattress pads and pillows, as well as sheets and blankets, need weekly hot washes to kill dust mites.

BUY THROW RUGS, NOT CARPETS: You can wash your rugs and get dust, pet dander, mold, and mites out, which you can't do with carpeting. If you don't want to redecorate, at the very least rent an industrial-strength carpet shampooer on a regular basis.

If you have severe and debilitating allergic reactions, or if you have ever experienced a mild anaphylactic shock, you should at once consult a physician who can prescribe an Epipen (filled with a self-injectable dose of epinephrine which will help you breathe until you can get to an emergency room). You may also be counseled to consider allergy desensitization, in which you receive injections of the offending allergens in gradually increasing doses. Reflexology and the other alternative treatments listed above can help you boost the immune system and reduce your sensitivity to allergens.

✳

ANEMIA

You've been weak and run-down, and you look awfully pale. Every once in a while you can hear your heart pounding, and there's a ringing in your ears. No matter how much rest you get, you're always ready to crawl into bed.

If you're anemic, you don't have enough red blood cells in your circulatory system, and those you have may not be producing enough hemoglobin, the pigment that carries oxygen in the red blood cells. The reason you feel so tired is that these cells aren't carrying enough oxygen to all parts of your body.

Anemia often stems from vitamin and mineral deficiencies, which may be caused by poor nutrition or chronic alcoholism (the alcoholic generally drinks his meals, so he isn't eating a proper diet). In this category are iron-deficiency anemia, folate-deficiency anemia, and pernicious anemia (inability to absorb vitamin B_{12}).

The condition may also stem from cancer or exposure to radiation. In aplastic anemia the bone marrow isn't manufacturing sufficient red cells to support the system.

Anemia may also result from losing a lot of blood through injury or trauma; bleeding ulcers can make you anemic, and some new mothers become anemic after giving birth.

Hemolytic anemias are caused by the destruction of red blood cells. These may be hereditary (like sickle-cell anemia) or may develop over time because of mismatched blood transfusions, drug allergies, cancer, or serious infections.

SYMPTOMS: Extreme fatigue, palpitations, shortness of

breath, headaches, loss of appetite, dizziness, ringing in the ears, burning tongue, and pale, clammy skin.

Areas to Treat/Types of Manipulation

Work both feet completely first. Then find the location of the spleen, and work that reflex carefully (see Chapter 3 for guidance):

Spleen: Apply gradual circular pressure with thumb tip and pad.

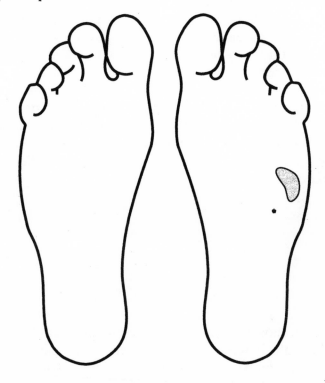

PREVENTIVE MEASURES AND COMPLEMENTARY TREATMENTS

Reflexology works well in conjunction with other alternative therapies and commonsense measures. For example:

START EATING RIGHT: You may need more protein than you've been getting. Start by swearing off junk food, and then plan your diet to include more red meat (with all the fat trimmed off), poultry without skin, fish, and legumes.

TAKE IRON: If your regular multivitamin doesn't include this mineral, it's important to supplement it with 30 mg. of iron daily.

SLEEP RIGHT: Try to get seven to eight hours of undisturbed sleep per night. During the deepest stages of sleep the body is able to restore and replenish its cells.

Reflexology can assist in the stimulation of new red cells. However, anemia should be treated by a physician who will do blood tests to determine the type and severity of the anemia and counsel you on the best diet and supplementation plan.

ANGINA PECTORIS

You are shoveling snow and suddenly get a painful tightening right in the middle of your chest, radiating out to your jaw and down your left arm. It gets so bad you put down the shovel. You feel anxious, clammy, terrified that you are going to die. This has to be a heart attack, doesn't it? But as soon as you rest, the pain goes away. Maybe you imagined it—but you probably didn't.

Angina pectoris (translated as "pain in the chest" and

sometimes called stable angina) is the sign that the heart is not getting enough oxygen because the arteries are too narrow to allow for continuous blood flow. When you rest, of course, the heart doesn't need as much oxygen, so the pain goes away. (Another type of angina, unstable angina, may occur even when you're not exerting yourself and doesn't diminish when you rest.)

Angina is a symptom of coronary artery disease, a condition in which fatty deposits called plaque have narrowed or blocked the arteries that carry blood to the heart. Most, but not all, people have had bouts of angina long before they ever have a heart attack. It is crucial that you pay attention to this warning signal; it could save your life by making you take steps to change your lifestyle and protect your heart.

SYMPTOMS: Angina is described by different people in different ways, but the Mayo Clinic offers the following adjectives so that you can distinguish angina from other types of chest pain. It may be "crushing, constricting, aching, squeezing, burning, strangling, like a gas pain, like an upper back ache, tight, cold, clammy, nauseating, full, heavy, or making you feel weak."

AREAS TO TREAT/TYPES OF MANIPULATION

Work both feet completely first. Then find the locations of reflexes that correspond to these organs, and work them in the following order (see Chapter 3 for guidance):

1. Heart: Using thumb tip, work around reflex with circular motion.
2. Adrenals: Apply direct pressure with thumb tip.
3. Bronchi: With the tip and edge of thumbs, glide from the base of the toes up toward the instep.

4. Lungs: With the tip and edge of thumbs, work up and down and left to right.

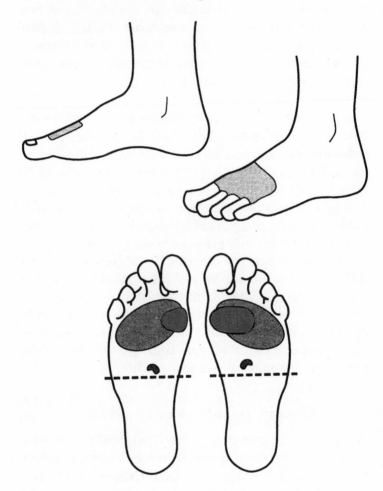

Preventive Measures and Complementary Treatments

Reflexology works well in conjunction with other alternative therapies and commonsense measures. For example:

MAINTAIN A VERY LOW-FAT DIET: Dr. Dean Ornish has

shown that a diet containing 10 percent fat can be one of the linchpins to getting the heart and circulatory system back in shape. An excellent diet lowers total cholesterol and triglycerides. If you are committed to clean arteries, you must eat nothing that walks, swims, flies, or crawls. There are many excellent heart-healthy cookbooks to help you get started.

GO OUT AND RUN: Or do any other form of aerobic exercise daily. Moderate regular activity has been shown to lower LDL cholesterol and raise HDL cholesterol. It also lowers blood pressure and heart rate and makes you feel wonderful, so that you'll be able to stick to your diet.

REDUCE YOUR STRESS: Stress can actually elevate LDL cholesterol and trigger the production of stress hormones that can make negative changes in the blood vessels. When you're overwhelmed with responsibility, pressure, anger, etc., your arteries constrict along with your muscles, preventing free circulation.

A regular program of meditation and breathing, yoga, or tai chi chuan can teach you to relax fully and handle distress as you enjoy the challenge of the pleasurable stresses (a promotion, a marriage, etc.) that make life worthwhile.

TRY AN HERB: Hawthorn has been used for cardiac problems for centuries. It is a vasodilator (it opens the blood vessels) and lowers blood pressure and cholesterol as it maximizes oxygen uptake during exercise. Motherwort (also known as lionheart) is also an excellent cardiac tonic. It supplies minerals, trace elements, and alkaloids to the heart. Either can be taken as an infusion (2 to 4 teaspoons of the dried herb infused in water) or as a tincture (15 to 25 drops, three times daily).

HOMEOPATHIC HELP: The remedies Nux vomica, Cactus, and Aurum muriaticum are recommended for angina.

Take 30C potency of Nux and Aurum; 3X of Cactus tincture.

Angina is one sign of a severe cardiac condition. You must see a doctor if you are having chest pains, whether or not you think they are significant. A physician will do a thorough workup, including an EKG and stress test, and may prescribe nitroglycerine tablets to be placed under the tongue when you have an angina attack. Reflexology and the alternative therapies listed above can reduce the pain of angina and help you develop a healthy lifestyle that may reverse heart disease.

ANXIETY

There's that lump in the pit of your stomach, and your hands are starting to shake. It's ridiculous, you know, but you just can't handle the dread inside you. You want to run away, but you think you can get a grip if you try. You just have to walk into your boss's office and take whatever he dishes out.

Anxiety is a state of apprehension about something that may be real or imaginary, a set of appropriate and inappropriate reactions that overlap and mix together. Generally anxiety creates a sense of dread and foreboding that is connected with a past unresolved event over which you may have current concerns.

A confrontation with an unleashed, snarling dog will cause fear, but the residue of feelings that arise every time you see or think about dogs is anxiety. If the dread becomes great enough, and the preparations to avoid that dread elaborate enough, you have a phobia. When you spend most of your time avoiding the fearful element, you have an obsessive-compulsive disorder. If repeated attempts to avoid the awful feelings fail, the experience may become so overwhelming as to cause panic. Your heartbeat escalates, your head pounds, and you feel you must escape—or you might die.

It doesn't take a vicious animal to cause anxiety, however; many people feel anxious on a daily basis without having any concrete trigger for their reaction. This free-floating anxiety is more difficult to treat than the type that relates to a real event or object.

SYMPTOMS: Feelings of dread, dry mouth, sweaty palms, palpitations, gastrointestinal upset. In addition, you may develop complex strategies (compulsions) to avoid the source of your anxiety (obsessions)—for example, crossing the street when a dog is walking toward you, repeatedly washing your hands to rid them of germs and bacteria, etc.

AREAS TO TREAT/TYPES OF MANIPULATION

Work both feet completely first. Then find the location of the solar plexus, and work that reflex carefully (see Chapter 3 for guidance):

Solar Plexus: With thumb tip, apply gradual pressure in the middle of reflex, and work out to the edges.

PREVENTIVE MEASURES AND COMPLEMENTARY TREATMENTS

Reflexology works well in conjunction with other alternative therapies and commonsense measures. For example:

BEHAVIOR CHANGE: A monitored program of behavior change and desensitization often works exceptionally well. You must be committed to "going through the fire"—that is, facing the object of your fear. If you are

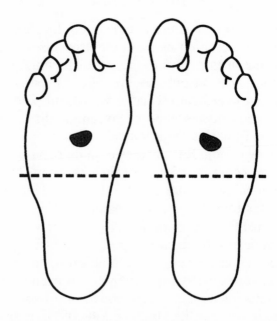

anxious about dogs, you would be given a picture of first a sweet puppy to look at, then a mature, strong dog, and finally an aggressive dog on a leash being controlled by his owner. Once you were comfortable with these interventions, you would be asked to stay at a considerable distance from a real dog, slowly and gradually closing the space between you over several sessions. Finally you would be asked to walk a dog on a leash, pet a dog, and get down on its level to look it in the eye.

TRY A FLOWER: The Bach flower remedy for anxiety is Rescue Remedy. Take 5 or 6 drops under the tongue or mixed with half a glass of water.

RELAX PROGRESSIVELY: This technique involves lying down and first tensing, then letting go of the muscles in each of your various body parts. Begin with the toes, curling them in tightly and then suddenly releasing the tension. Move on to your feet, ankles, calves, knees, thighs, pelvic area, lower back, waist, chest, mid-back, upper back, head (including the chin, jaw, nose, mouth, forehead, and scalp), neck, shoulders, forearms, wrists, and fingers. As you tense and release each body part, think about letting go of the feelings and fears you have and releasing them into the air.

BREATHE DEEPLY: When we're frightened, we typically start to breathe from the upper chest and mouth. In order to calm the mind, we can center the body by bringing the breath down to the diaphragm and belly. Start by lying on your back and putting your hands over the point in the center of your abdomen, about three inches down from your waistband. Inhale, letting the breath push your abdomen up against your hands; exhale, and let the abdomen relax. Consciously try to keep the breath out of your neck and chest region; don't worry, the lungs will expand on their own. Once you feel comfortable on your back, try the diaphragmatic breathing seated and standing, then walking. When you inhale, you are taking in oxygen and energy to combat your anxieties; when you exhale, you are letting out carbon dioxide and the residual fears that have plagued you.

INHALE AN HERB: Aromatherapy, with or without massage, can reduce some of the dread you're feeling. Try marjoram, rosewood, ylang-ylang, or sandalwood oil mixed with a carrier oil in a defuser by your bed at night, or ask a friend to give you a massage with it.

If reflexology and the other alternative treatments listed above have not alleviated your anxiety, and your symptoms are interfering with your daily functioning, you may wish to consult a physician for traditional psychotherapy or medical (mood-altering drug) intervention.

ARTHRITIS

The first time you couldn't open a jar, you worried. But when you felt so crippled up you couldn't hold your grandchild's hand without pain, you were seriously concerned. Everything, from your hands to your hips and knees, seems to ache all the time, and wet weather makes it even worse.

"Arthritis" is a catchall term for nearly a hundred rheumatic diseases—that is, conditions that affect the joints, inflaming them so that they are swollen and painful. One in seven people suffers from one of these conditions.

Osteoarthritis is a condition in which the cartilage that cushions the joints and bones is worn away, leaving no padding at the ends of the bones. This erosion causes the bones to rub together, making them swollen and painful. Rheumatoid arthritis affects the connective tissue, so that the lining of the joint (the synovial membrane) becomes inflamed, and the inflammation destroys the cartilage. As scar tissue takes the place of the cartilage, the joint becomes swollen and rigid.

Other joint diseases in the arthritis family are gout, spinal arthritis, psoriatic arthritis, juvenile arthritis, ankylosing spondylitis, bursitis/tendonitis, carpal tunnel syndrome, fibromyalgia, and lupus. Reflexology treatments for any and all of these conditions may help rebalance energy flowing to the joints and thus alleviate pain.

One of my clients, who had had surgery on her shoulder six years earlier, developed arthritis in the shoulder and neck. Her doctor put her on medication, but it did nothing for her. In my first treatment I worked on her neck and shoulder reflex points, her kidneys and adrenals, her ileocecal valve, and her spine. She had almost immediate pain relief and increased mobility both during and after treatment, which we continued on a biweekly basis.

SYMPTOMS: Aching, pain, swelling, tenderness, and redness in one or several joints as well as stiffness or restriction of movement in joints. Damp weather can exacerbate these problems. Very often those with rheumatoid arthritis develop fever and fatigue, which may appear and reappear for no obvious reason.

AREAS TO TREAT/TYPES OF MANIPULATION

Work both feet completely first. Then find the locations of reflexes that correspond to these organs, and work them in the following order (see Chapter 3 for guidance):

1. Kidneys: Apply direct pressure with thumb tip.
2. Adrenals: Apply direct pressure with thumb tip.
3. Solar Plexus: With thumb tip, apply gradual pressure in the middle of the reflex and work out to the edges.

PREVENTIVE MEASURES AND COMPLEMENTARY TREATMENTS

Reflexology works well in conjunction with other alternative therapies and commonsense measures. For example:

LOSE WEIGHT IF YOU HAVE TO: The less pressure on knees, hips, ankles, and feet, the less pain they'll feel. If you're thinner, you place less stress on your joints and therefore may be able to slow the process of cartilage erosion.

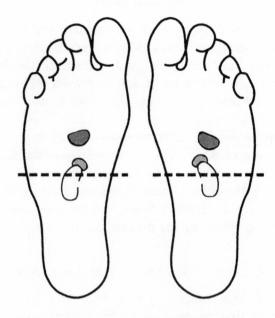

GET SOME REST: Know your limitations. If you are really in pain, you shouldn't push yourself. Instead be certain to get at least seven hours' sleep at night, and take an hour during the day to sit or lie down quietly and perhaps visualize the pain slowly dissolving like an Alka-Seltzer in water. See the bubbles bursting from the source, and imagine them as pain molecules breaking off from your body and leaving you feeling whole and well.

GO OUT AND EXERCISE: Moderate exercise, such as walking, swimming, bicycling, dancing, and skiing, will increase endurance. Yoga and tai chi chuan train the body to be flexible and elastic. All these forms of activity will stabilize weak joints and improve function.

PROTECT YOUR JOINTS: Various different braces and devices are available to cover and protect knees, wrists, shoulders, and other joints. Most are available in pharmacies and supermarkets. There are also occupational tools you can buy—bent forks and spoons that are easier to hold than conventional ones, jar and doorknob openers, etc.—that may make life easier.

USE HEAT AND COLD: An ice pack is usually the first line of treatment for pain, because it shrinks the inflamed tissue. Arthritis usually responds better to cold than heat, although a warm bath or whirlpool every once in a while may help loosen stiff joints.

TAKE IBUPROFEN AS NEEDED: Nonsteroidal anti-inflammatory drugs (NSAIDs) will slow the body's production of prostaglandins, hormonelike fatty acids that play a part in pain and inflammation. They don't upset the stomach like aspirin but should not be overused. Consult a physician about appropriate dosage if you need to take ibuprofen or other NSAIDs daily.

If neither reflexology nor any of the alternative treatments listed above provide relief, you should consult a physician who will do a thorough workup, including X rays and blood tests, and may prescribe cortisone and other medications that can be helpful.

ASTHMA

You inhale, but only a thin ribbon of oxygen enters your nose and mouth. You are gasping like a fish out of water, and you feel desperate; perhaps you will never get a full breath.

Asthma is a chronic condition of the lungs in which the bronchial tubes leading from the trachea (the windpipe) to the lungs are severely narrowed as the result of the contraction of the muscles lining them. When the tubes close up, it's more difficult for you to get oxygen in and particularly hard for you to get carbon dioxide out. For this reason, asthmatics usually inhale with short gasps and exhale with long wheezes. The air hunger caused by this condition can make you panicky and terrified that your lungs will close up entirely.

Asthma stems from a variety of causes, from air pollution to emotional upset. We all are bombarded with a variety of foreign substances in the air, but most individuals react with a sneeze that clears the respiratory system of this invader. An asthmatic, on the other hand, is so highly sensitive to many elements that he fights back by producing antibodies (disease fighters) no matter how benign the substance he's breathing. His cells release stress-related chemicals that cause the bronchial tubes to close up. Extreme sensitivity to anything in the environment—pollen, cat dander, or a fight with the boss—can set up an almost continual supply of these damaging chemicals. Although it's commonly thought that people get asthmatic reactions only at certain times of the year, when pollens, molds, or spores are rampant, true asthmatics will feel miserable all year from inhaling microscopic house mites or being subject to pet fur and dander, tobacco smoke, paint fumes, car exhaust, air pollutants, and various foods, preservatives, and such medicines as penicillin, vaccines, and anesthetics.

Asthma is typically treated with bronchodilators, drugs that widen the bronchial tubes and allow more air to come through. If you need to take this medication, your doctor will prescribe an inhaler that you carry with you and use as needed. It's important not to overuse this medication and to become aware of increasing need, which would indicate that your condition is getting worse.

Stress is also a cause of asthmatic attacks. Many physicians believe that having a hair-trigger response to every little thing in the environment eventually lowers the immune system, making the individual more susceptible to illness.

The only boon to stress-related asthmatic attacks is that when we're panicked and feel a desire either to fight or to flee, our adrenal glands produce a stress hormone known as adrenaline. Adrenaline helps open the bronchial tubes so that it's easier to breathe. You'll note that the adrenal glands (where adrenaline is secreted) are key reflex points to treat for asthma; they balance the endocrine and the respiratory systems, both of which are necessary to prevent and treat asthma.

SYMPTOMS: Sudden shortness of breath and wheezing, occasionally accompanied by coughing. Asthmatics tend to be prone to chest infections because they can't clear their lungs fully and may store phlegm instead of expelling it. The onset of symptoms is often, but not always, triggered by a change of season and new irritations from spring, summer, and fall weeds, pollens, and fungal spores.

AREAS TO TREAT/TYPES OF MANIPULATION

Work both feet completely first. Then find the locations of reflexes that correspond to these organs, and work them in the following order (see Chapter 3 for guidance):

1. Bronchi: With the tip and edge of thumbs, glide from the base of the toes up toward the instep.
2. Lungs: With the tip and edge of thumb, work up and down and left to right.
3. Solar Plexus: With the thumb tip, apply gradual pressure in the middle of the reflex and work out to edges.
4. Adrenals: Apply direct pressure with thumb tip.

5. Ileocecal Valve: Apply direct pressure with thumb tip.

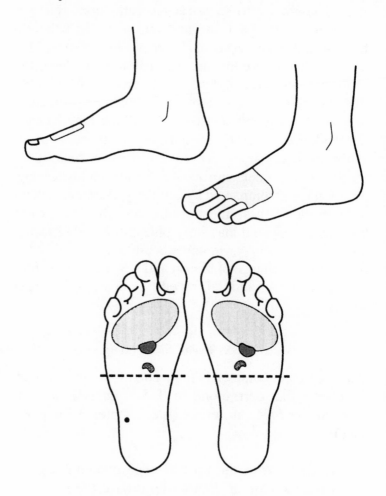

PREVENTIVE MEASURES AND COMPLEMENTARY TREATMENTS

Reflexology works well in conjunction with other alternative therapies and commonsense measures. For example:

STAY AWAY FROM SMOKE: Tobacco smoke can bring on

an attack, so stay in smoke-free areas as much as you can. Wood smoke is also a problem, so avoid cozy winter fireplaces.

LEARN YOUR FOOD ALLERGIES: You can test yourself on the most common foods that cause allergic reactions to find out if there are items you should eliminate from your diet. (If you get severe attacks, don't experiment with these foods; simply don't eat them.) Start with milk, eggs, nuts, seafood, and wheat products, the most common offenders.

ELIMINATE ADDITIVES: Food additives such as MSG and sulfites that keep foods fresh can trigger asthma attacks. Be sure you ask what's in the foods you eat in restaurants or takeout places and avoid these chemicals.

TRY A CUP OF COFFEE: Caffeine, which gives a surge of adrenaline similar to several drugs used to treat asthma, can open your airways in a pinch. Take two cups of coffee, cocoa, soda, or tea, or eat two chocolate bars if you are having trouble. Be sure to eat or drink slowly, giving yourself time to recover between bites or sips.

EXERCISE AND BREATHE: Swimming is the perfect exercise for an asthmatic since the throat is kept moist in all that water, and a dry throat often triggers an asthma attack. If you're working on land—jogging, walking, biking, or doing any other aerobic activity—be sure to breathe with your mouth closed so as not to dry out the back of your throat.

If you have asthma, you must be under a physician's care and will probably need to carry an inhaler. Reflexology and the above complementary treatments will provide a certain amount of relief and may help you cut down on your medication dosage and frequency.

⁎

Back Problems

"Oh, my aching back!" This is one of the most common complaints of people over forty, although back problems can occur at any age. You move funny, and it hits you like a jackhammer; you lift a leg to get out of bed and find you're stuck half in and half out, in agony from head to toe.

Before you can understand what causes the back to ache, it's important to know some basic landmarks. The back is composed of thirty-three vertebrae: seven cervical (neck), twelve thoracic (rib), five lumbar (below the curve of the waist), and five fused vertebrae (the sacrum, your "sit" bones) and the coccyx (five small vertebrae that make up the "tailbone"). These structures are separated by cushioned disks that circle the spinal cord. Nerves and blood vessels form an intricate network that passes in and out of the disks and cord.

At each end of the spinal column is a supportive structure that attaches to the limbs; the pectoral girdle holds the arms in place, and the pelvic girdle holds the legs in place.

The most common form of backache is caused by a misalignment of the vertebrae, which chiropractors and osteopathic physicians refer to as a subluxation. An injury or overuse of any part of the spine can cause damage, which may begin as a tearing of ligaments, an inflammation of the disks, or a combination of these two conditions. Pressure on the disks means pressure on the nerves, which of course produces pain. The longer this irritation persists, the more the pressure placed on the traumatized areas, and the more we try to compensate by holding ourselves still or moving differently. If the area is very badly damaged, the entire disk may slip out of place or become pinched between two vertebrae and rupture.

Disks age along with the body and may wear down and develop painful bony growths over time with incorrect movement. The thinner they become, the less protection the spine has.

It's not just the disks that get older, of course, but the bone itself. Osteoporosis, a disease in which the interior of the bone loses mass and density, is common in women after menopause and in elderly men and women. When the increasingly demineralized spine can no longer support the upright structure of the body, the back may bow in the classic "dowager's hump," and as a result, the entire thoracic cavity may come to rest on the pelvic girdle, causing a great deal of pain.

One of my clients, Angela, who suffered from lower back pain and sciatica for years, finally got tired of pain medication and asked if reflexology might help. Because she'd had this problem so long, we worked intensively, three times a week at first, on her spine reflexes as well as her shoulder, hip, and knee points, and on her kidneys and adrenals to help reduce inflammation. After her first treatment she said she could feel a change; by the time we'd been together for three weeks, her back pain was so greatly reduced she was able to begin an exercise program. She continued to treat herself and now swims and walks several times a week.

SYMPTOMS: Different symptoms will indicate different types of back disorders. All pain described may range from mildly annoying to excruciating, and some may make walking or even turning over difficult or impossible.

Sciatica: A dull ache that runs from the center of the

buttock down one leg (it can be present on both sides). Sciatica can be mild or extremely painful and severe.

Lumbago: Usually the pain stays in the lumbar region, but it can spread to the buttocks and thighs. The pain is usually worse with bending, straightening up, or any side-to-side movement.

Slipped Disk: The onset of this sharp pain shooting through the back usually comes with a difficult or awkward movement. It is sometimes described as "feeling the back go or give out." Coughing or sneezing may leave you in agony.

Arthritis: Stiffness as well as a lessening of flexibility is common. Pain usually starts lower down on both sides, and as the spine begins to fuse together over time, the pain increases.

Fractured Vertebra: This results in a localized constant pain that is worse with any type of movement.

Gallstones: These can cause pain just below the right ribs in the front and back. They may be accompanied by nausea.

Shingles: The same pain as gallstones; however, a blistering rash appears after a few days.

Pain During Pregnancy: This is usually an ache in the lower lumbar region, caused by pressure of the growing fetus.

Areas to Treat/Types of Manipulation

Work both feet completely first. Then find the locations of reflexes for the spine (see Chapter 3 for guidance). Working the spine alone will help the various symptoms of back pain, although they are quite different. Obviously, if you are also having pain in the neck, shoulders, or other areas, refer to those organs in Chapter 3, and work them as well.

1. Spine: Holding the foot with one hand, glide the other thumb tip from top to bottom of reflex. Make sure that you concentrate on the area that most closely corresponds to the part of your back that is affected.
2. Kidneys: Apply direct pressure with thumb tip.
3. Adrenals: Apply direct pressure with thumb tip.
4. Solar Plexus: With thumb tip, apply gradual pressure in the middle of the reflex, and work out to the edges.

PREVENTIVE MEASURES AND COMPLEMENTARY TREATMENTS

Reflexology works well in conjunction with other alternative therapies and commonsense measures. For example:

CONSIDER R.I.C.E.: Most professionals suggest that you rest the back, use ice, compress the area (you can use a belt or back brace), and elevate the area.

STRETCH AND TONE: For preventive care and also in treatment for a bad back, nothing beats the daily stretching of your muscles and ligaments. Right after you wake up, if you've been sitting at a desk or in a car for hours, or any time you feel stiff, stretch slowly up, down, and side to side. Do this slowly and carefully, avoiding movements that overextend your muscles.

DON'T LIFT: Whenever possible, get someone else to lift heavy objects, shovel snow, or open sash windows. If you must lift, *always* bend your knees.

EXERCISE WHEN READY: After a couple of days of bed rest for acute pain, it's time to get up and move a little. Try lying flat on the floor and pulling your knees into your chest; when that's tolerable, you can begin to rock back and forth and side to side in this position. Swimming—which is great preventive care for your back—is also an excellent activity as you're recuperating.

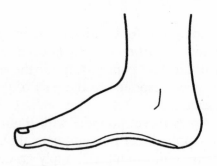

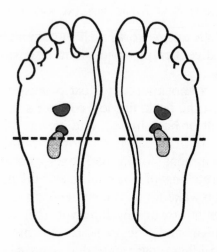

SLEEP RIGHT: Most chiropractors and osteopaths recommend sleeping on your side in an S curve, with your knees tucked into your chest. Under no circumstances should you sleep on your stomach, which gets the neck and back out of alignment.

STAND UP STRAIGHT: Good posture can make a huge difference in the way your back feels. Stand in front of a mirror, and be sure your head is erect, in line with your neck and upper back. Your shoulders should be sloped downward but not hunched forward or backward, and your pelvis should relax down; you can accomplish this by standing against a wall and trying to push your waist up against it.

ASPIRIN RELIEF: One aspirin or ibuprofen a day can reduce swelling and inflammation in your back and take away the pain.

GET SOME SUPPORT: Whether you're driving, sitting at a computer, or sleeping, back supports are excellent for prevention and treatment of pain. Most supermarkets and drugstores carry lumbar devices you can use at home and at work; you may also want to get a chiropractor-approved mattress or put a board under the mattress you now own.

TAI CHI CHUAN FOR THE SPINE: The ancient Chinese moving meditation known as tai chi chuan creates a "supple spine," which is described in classic texts as "an iron bar wrapped in cotton" and a "string of pearls." The fluid tai chi chuan "forms," which you can learn from a tape, a book, or a class, will realign your vertebrae gently, strengthening the spine and surrounding muscles.

If none of the above measures provides relief and if you have been in pain for days—particularly if the back pain is accompanied by chest pain, stomach cramps, or fever—consult a physician.

Bladder Problems (see also Prostate Problems, p. 243, and Urinary Tract Infections, p. 285)

That burning, painful feeling when you urinate is excruciating. Or perhaps you just relieved yourself, and now you have to go again. There are times when you don't think you'll make it to the toilet in time and other times when you find it impossible to start the flow. And you are never so embarrassed as when you sneeze or cough and find that you've wet your pants a little. Is it nerves? Somehow, you don't think so, but the problem is too embarrassing to discuss with anyone.

Both men and women may occasionally suffer from a variety of bladder problems, and with increasing age, as the musculature around the urethra and the various organs in the pelvic cavity become less elastic, the problem may become chronic.

The most common difficulty with the bladder is an infection caused by *E. coli* bacteria, which occur naturally in the vagina, migrate to the urethra, and irritate the bladder wall. The best way to deal with this problem is to flush the invaders out—by drinking and voiding as often as you can.

Many people think that a dysfunctional bladder is too awful a subject to talk about, but it's important to discuss these problems with a physician when they first appear, because early, aggressive treatment is enormously successful. In addition to reflexology, there are many natural ways to treat bladder problems.

SYMPTOMS: Various troubles that you may encounter will have different symptoms. They include:

Bladder Infections: A desperate urge to urinate, but difficulty with the flow. A burning sensation while urinating.

Urge and Stress Incontinence: These problems are most common in postmenopausal women and the elderly. With urge incontinence, you have an urgent need to urinate frequently, even after you have just voided. With stress incontinence, you may leak some urine when you cough, sneeze, laugh, have an orgasm, or change position.

Kidney Failure: You will note a reduction in the volume of urine. The urine may be cloudy or tinged with blood. You may also have a lot of swelling in the feet, hands, and around the eyes. In addition, you may be dizzy and fatigued much of the time and have chronic nausea, diarrhea, dry skin, and difficulty in breathing.

Bladder Cancer: You may have blood in the urine or frequent, difficult, or painful urination.

IN WOMEN: Cystocele: You may have a predisposition to this condition if it runs in your family. Repeated difficult births can also create a cystocele. If the bladder drops and protrudes into the vagina, you may feel a fullness in the vaginal area and find it difficult to urinate.

IN MEN: Prostatitis (inflammation of the prostate gland): You may have trouble starting the flow of urine, reduced force in urinating and dribbling at the end of the flow, increased frequency of urge, or burning sensation while urinating. In addition, you may have an aching lower back, fever, and chills.

Areas to Treat/Types of Manipulation

Work both feet completely first. Then find the locations of the reflexes corresponding to these organs, and work them in the following order (see Chapter 3 for guidance):

1. Bladder: Apply circular pressure with thumb pad.
2. Kidneys: Apply direct pressure with thumb tip.
3. Ureter: Glide thumb tip down ureter from kidney to bladder.

Preventive Measures and Complementary Treatments

Reflexology works well in conjunction with other alternative therapies and commonsense measures. For example:

DRINK CRANBERRY OR CHERRY JUICE: Both these juices contain quinolinic acid, which converts to hippuric acid in the liver, as well as vitamin C. These have been shown to have a positive effect in some women in combating the infection.

DRINK TO YOUR HEART'S CONTENT: Plain springwater will flush the kidneys and urethra. Try to keep a water bottle or glass by your side throughout the day and keep sipping. Void at least once an hour. The more you hold your urine, the more bacteria collect in the bladder, and the longer you keep the infection active.

VOID AFTER INTERCOURSE: Since the penis can push the bacteria from the vagina into the bladder, it's a good idea to go to the bathroom after sexual activity. For the same reason, you might want to switch from tampons to sanitary pads when you have your period.

TAKE A HOT BATH: The warm water can be very soothing to your urinary tract and can alleviate the burning, stinging pain you feel as you void.

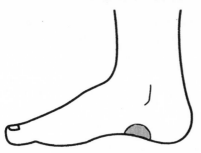

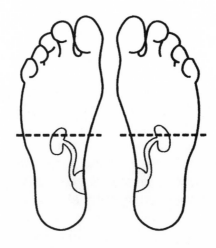

TRY NSAIDS: Nonsteroidal anti-inflammatory drugs, such as ibuprofen, can reduce the inflammation of your infection.

A simple bladder infection will respond well to reflexology and the alternative therapies listed above. If you are still having symptoms after a week of these treatments, or if your symptoms include blood in the urine, fever, nausea, vomiting, or severe lower back pain, they may stem from a more serious condition, which should be diagnosed by a medical practitioner who will do an examination and conduct laboratory tests that will reveal the source of your problem.

BLEEDING GUMS (GINGIVITIS)

When you brush your teeth, your toothbrush looks as if you have dipped it in red paint. Your gums are swollen and tender, and it's impossible to floss without bringing on a flow.

Bleeding gums, also known as gingivitis, are the first stage of periodontal disease, in which the gums become swollen and infected and bleed easily. Gum disease, which is the major cause of tooth loss, can be prevented by keeping the mouth clear of plaque, bacteria, and food deposits and by maintaining any tooth prostheses, such as crowns, fillings, or dentures, in good condition.

Bleeding gums may also stem from a nutritional deficiency, scurvy, caused by a lack of vitamin C. Gingivitis is also a common problem of people with HIV infection and other diseases in which the immune system is severely compromised. The blood vessels become fragile and easily bruised.

SYMPTOMS: Swollen, painful gums, bad breath, tooth loss.

Any activity in the mouth, from toothbrushing to French kissing, may bring on a flow of blood. The gums are sore and tender, and flossing can be painful.

AREAS TO TREAT/TYPES OF MANIPULATION

Work both feet completely first. Then find the locations of the reflexes that correspond to these organs, and work them in this order (see Chapter 3 for guidance):

1. Head: Using thumb tip, work the tips of the toes using a circular motion; then work all around the whole toe. Concentrate on the tops of the toes near the nails, which correspond to the teeth and gums.
2. Adrenals: Apply direct pressure with thumb tip.
3. Spleen: Apply gradual circular pressure with thumb tip and pad.

PREVENTIVE MEASURES AND COMPLEMENTARY TREATMENTS

Reflexology works well in conjunction with other alternative therapies and commonsense measures. For example:

MAINTAIN GOOD DENTAL HEALTH: Be sure to brush and floss twice daily. There are special rinses and mouthwashes that provide additional protection to your gums and teeth.

SUPPLEMENT YOUR MEALS: Pay attention to your vitamins and minerals. You should be taking 500–1,000 mg. of vitamin C daily in addition to a good multivitamin. You may also wish to supplement the B vitamins (at least 50 mg. daily to combat stress) and zinc (30 mg. daily to boost the immune system and prevent infection of the gums).

TAKE SOME HERBS: Echinacea and goldenseal are two herbs (often packaged together) that will boost your immune system.

SOOTHE THE PAIN: Apply oil of cloves to the gum area to provide relief from the soreness.

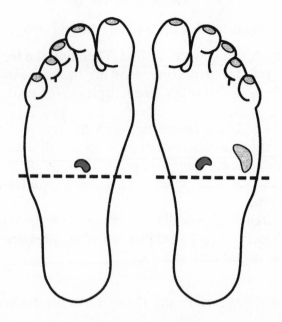

Reflexology and the other alternative therapies listed above will help your gums. However, you should see a dentist twice yearly for a prophylactic cleaning and checkup.

Blood Pressure, High
See Hypertension

Bronchitis

It seems as if that cold just hangs on and on, and you're well enough to go out, but you really feel miserable. You don't sleep well at night because you get this tickle in your throat that starts you coughing your head off and bringing up phlegm. During the day you're always short of breath, and it feels as though a weight were sitting on your chest.

Bronchitis is a persistent inflammation and thickening of the lining of the bronchial passages that cause an obstruction in the outflow of air. As the mucous membranes become irritated, they produce more mucus, and as it further clogs the already swollen airways, it becomes more difficult to breathe. You feel as though you must get the mucus up and out of your system, which gives you a productive cough. Many smokers have chronic bronchitis, but it may also be a by-product of a bad cold, during which time the bronchial tubes may have become irritated. It is usually caused by a virus (which means that antibiotics won't help), but it can also have a bacterial basis (medication can provide some relief).

SYMPTOMS: Chronic, productive cough (mucus may be yellowish green) and shortness of breath. Acute bronchitis is characterized by a foul-smelling sputum and is often confused with pneumonia. Untreated bronchitis may result in severe lung damage, which may bring on other respiratory diseases (chronic obstructive pulmonary disease, or COPD).

AREAS TO TREAT/TYPES OF MANIPULATION

Work both feet completely first. Then find the locations of the reflexes that correspond to these organs, and work them in the following order (see Chapter 3 for guidance):

1. Lungs: With tip and edge of thumb, work up and down and left to right.

2. Bronchi: With tip and edge of thumbs, glide from bases of toes down toward instep.
3. Solar Plexus: With thumb tip, apply gradual pressure in the middle of the reflex, and work out to the edges.
4. Spleen: Apply gradual circular pressure with thumb tip and pad.
5. Ileocecal Valve: Apply direct pressure with thumb tip.

Preventive Measures and Complementary Treatments

Reflexology works well in conjunction with other alternative therapies and commonsense measures. For example:

STOP SMOKING: This is the most important thing you can do for your lungs (and for the lungs of everyone around you!).

STEAM YOURSELF: Getting warm, moist air on the lungs is important to loosen the secretions in your chest and help bring them up. Make yourself a pot of herb tea (chamomile or Traditional Medicina's brand, Breathe Easy tea), and drape a towel over your head as you sit over the basin. You can also spend some time in a hot shower and remain in the bathroom with the door shut after you've finished bathing to take advantage of the steam.

DRINK FLUIDS: Pure springwater, herbal tea, and juices will help you water down the mucus and make it easier to bring up. Don't drink caffeinated beverages or alcohol, which actually dehydrate you by making you urinate more copiously and frequently.

AVOID COUGH SUPPRESSANTS: The idea is to get the mucus out out of your lungs rather than keep it down there. Unless your physician has prescribed a particular drug for you, stay away from cough medicine.

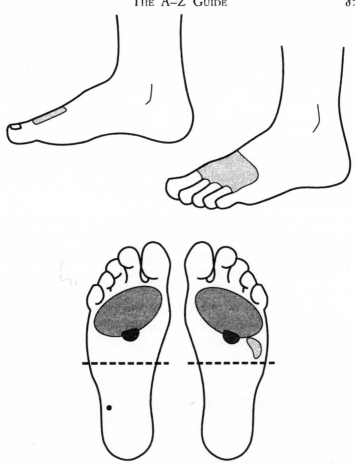

Bronchitis can be a serious condition if untreated. Reflexology and the alternative therapies listed above will alleviate the symptoms and balance the energy in the respiratory system so that it's easier for you to breathe. However, you should consult a physician if you've been coughing for more than two weeks and are still bringing up colored sputum or blood.

BURSITIS

You've been scrubbing floors all your life, and all of a sudden getting down in the position is excruciating. You can hardly bend your leg, and the knee is tender to the touch; it looks swollen and inflamed.

The bursas are small, fluid-filled pouches—eight around each shoulder, eleven around each knee, about seventy-eight on either side of the body—that absorb the shock of joint movement and cut down on the friction between bones, muscles, and ligaments. But these pouches are easily inflamed by infection or injury, either a sudden, one-time event or continual pressure on the area. "Housemaid's knee," "tennis elbow," and "one-side shoulder-bag tenderness" are common varieties of bursitis.

If you bang your elbow or ankle, for example, the membrane that lines the bursa will start producing more fluid, and consequently, the area will swell up and lose flexibility.

SYMPTOMS: Swelling and fluid around the large joints of the body, such as the shoulder, elbow, ankle, or knee. Occasionally bursitis will appear as a bunion at the joint between the big toe and the foot. The swelling may be so severe that it becomes impossible to move the joint.

AREAS TO TREAT/TYPES OF MANIPULATION

Work both feet completely first. Then find the locations of the reflexes that correspond to these organs, and work them in the following order (see Chapter 3 for guidance):

1. Shoulder: Apply firm circular pressure to reflex with thumb tip.
2. Adrenals: Apply direct pressure with thumb tip.

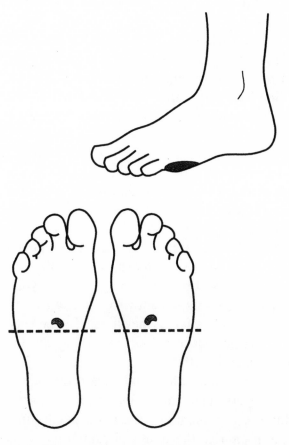

PREVENTIVE MEASURES AND COMPLEMENTARY TREATMENTS

Reflexology works well in conjunction with other alternative therapies and commonsense measures. For example:

DON'T USE IT IF IT HURTS: Repeated irritation of the affected joint only makes it worse. Take a rest from kneeling, hitting tennis balls, or wearing your shoulder bag (or any other activity that uses the joint).

WRAP IT UP: Immobilizing the area—wearing a sling or using crutches—is a more dramatic way to rest the area. This will give the joint a break and allow the swelling to come down.

APPLY ICE, THEN MOIST HEAT: Start by icing the area, especially if the joint is hot when you touch it. Switch to a heat pack or a warm, moist washcloth after ten minutes, then back to ice after ten more minutes. The alternating temperatures may alleviate some of the discomfort.

USE CASTOR OIL WITH HEAT: Once the joint is on the road to recovery and the swelling has gone down enough so that you can move it, rub the area with castor oil, cover it with a piece of flannel or wool, and then put a heating pad over it.

EXPERIMENT WITH RANGE OF MOTION: Although you don't want to use the joint too much, it's beneficial to move the area a little so that it doesn't get stiff. If your shoulder is painful, swing it gently in a circle or walk your fingers up a wall as far as they'll go. If your knee hurts, sit in a straight-backed chair and swing the lower leg gently back and forth.

TRY NSAIDS: Ibuprofen and other over-the-counter pain relievers may do some good; however, you shouldn't rely on them in order to be able to function. If you are in pain all the time and cannot move the joint, it's time to call your doctor.

If reflexology and the other alternative treatments provide no relief of your bursitis, consult a physician, who may recommend a short course of corticosteroid drugs or even complete bed rest to take pressure off the affected area.

CATARACTS

You can't see. At first it was just cloudy, and if you blinked, you could make out what was in front of you. But one day you woke up and looking through that one eye was like looking through pouring water. The image in front of you was blurred, as though broken into a thousand pieces.

A cataract is a thickening of coagulated proteins of which the lens of the eye is made. It is due partly to the aging process; as wild chemical reactants known as free radicals attach to normal cells, they can oxidize and harden the proteins within. Cataracts also occur because of disease (babies of mothers who contract German measles and individuals with diabetes, detached retinas, or glaucoma may develop cataracts). Other causes are metabolic disorders, vitamin-deficiency diseases, and high exposure to radiation.

The process of the development of the cataract is slow and insidious. At first there may be a slight clouding of the lens that impairs vision slightly. Over time the image seems broken up (as light is able to penetrate only in certain places), and finally the eye is able to pick up only the direction from which a light is aimed.

A cataract must be well developed, or mature, in order to be ripe enough to remove. This is accomplished surgically, usually with a laser treatment or an ultrasonic procedure that breaks up the cataract so that it can be vacuumed out of the eye. Very often a synthetic implant is inserted to replace the original lens. Other solutions are corrective eyeglasses or contact lenses.

SYMPTOMS: An inability to see clearly, usually out of only one eye. The individual will perceive glare in most

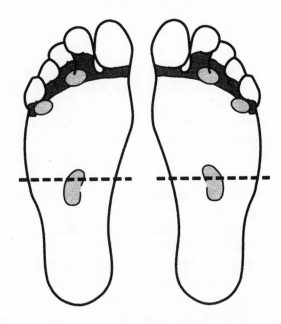

surroundings (because the affected lens scatters light instead of focusing it). When the cataract is ripe, it appears to be a milky white disk covering the center of the eye.

AREAS TO TREAT/TYPES OF MANIPULATION

Work both feet completely first. Then find locations of reflexes that correspond to these organs, and work them in the following order (see Chapter 3 for guidance):

1. Eye/Ear: Apply direct circular pressure with thumb tip.
2. Kidneys: Apply direct pressure with thumb tip.
3. Neck: Using thumb and index finger, manipulate "necks" of toes thoroughly.

Cataracts can cause blindness. If you are having difficulty seeing, you should have a full exam by an optometrist or an ophthalmologist. If you do have a cataract, you may have to wait until it is ripe to have it removed, and during that time, reflexology can help balance energy in the eye to make vision slightly clearer.

COLITIS

You love vegetables, but they don't love you. Some days it doesn't matter what you eat: You get a pain in the lower abdomen, and your stool has traces of blood and mucus. You may have diarrhea several times a day, on awakening and right after each meal.

Colitis, or an inflammation of the colon, may be due to a bacterial infection or to several other diseases, including irritable bowel, Crohn's disease, or amebiasis. It tends to be chronic and to recur even after it's cleared up, and it can make figuring out which foods will be most easily digestible quite difficult.

Using reflexology, I've been able to restore better digestive function for several clients over the years. John had terrible problems with vegetables, especially when he ate them raw in a salad. I concentrated work on his stomach, the entire colon, and his small intestine. Only two days after his first treatment, he felt so much better he ate his first green salad in months, with no ill effects. He was so excited about reflexology he wanted to continue working on himself. I showed him the points he had to concentrate on, and he's been fine since.

SYMPTOMS: An irritable bowel with a variety of conflicting symptoms, including both diarrhea and constipation, sometimes accompanied by abdominal cramps and traces of blood or mucus in the stool. Often the individual will feel a desperate need to void the bowel first thing in the morning as well as during or after meals. Gas, bloating, nausea, headache, and fatigue may also deplete the energy of the sufferer.

Areas to Treat/Types of Manipulation

Work both feet completely first. Then find locations of reflexes that correspond to these organs, and work them in the following order (see Chapter 3 for guidance):

1. Colon: Beginning on the right foot, glide the thumb tip from the ileocecal valve up the ascending colon, across the transverse colon, to the inside edge of the foot.

    Continue with the left foot. Glide the thumb left to right across the transverse colon, down the descending colon, and end with a slight upward hook.
2. Solar Plexus: With the thumb tip, apply gradual pressure in the middle of the reflex, and work out to the edges.
3. Adrenals: Apply direct pressure with thumb tip.

Preventive Measures and Complementary Treatments

Reflexology works well in conjunction with other alternative therapies and commonsense measures. For example:

DON'T OVERDO: If you are aware that certain foods may set off a bout of colitis, refrain from eating them, or eat only small portions.

GIVE UP MILK: It is possible that your colitis is caused by a lactose intolerance. You might want to experiment with removing milk products from your diet and switching to Lactaid, a lactose-reduced or -removed milk.

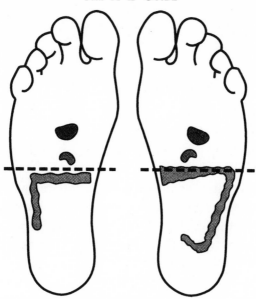

RUN AROUND: Exercise can often promote good bowel action and is also helpful in promoting general physical and emotional health. A daily walk, swim, or bike ride may help you digest food more completely and more easily.

CALM DOWN: Anxiety can often cause an irritable bowel. The digestive tract contains a secondary nervous system (the enteric nervous system) that can produce the butterflies in the stomach and cramps typical of colitis. A regular program of meditation and visualization, yoga, or tai chi chuan will teach you to breathe fully and easily and give you the emotional tools to settle an upset stomach.

If reflexology and the alternative treatments listed above do not alleviate the symptoms of your colitis, you should see your physician for a full workup and diagnostic tests to rule out more serious conditions like ulcerative colitis.

Conjunctivitis

The picture in the mirror isn't pretty. You look as if you've been up for weeks. Your eye is red and weepy, perfectly disgusting.

Conjunctivitis, or pinkeye, is an inflammation of the conjunctiva, the mucous membrane that lines the inner surface of the eyelid. If the condition is caused by a virus or a foreign body in the eye (as little as an eyelash can do it), only one eye will be affected; if the cause is an allergy or a bacterial infection or a swim in a contaminated pool or lake, generally both eyes will be red.

Conjunctivitis is highly contagious. If you touch your eye, then touch someone else, and that person touches his eye, he will probably get it. It is common in children and may be an additional symptom to measles. Very often schools insist that parents keep children with conjunctivitis home until it clears up.

SYMPTOMS: A red, watery eye or eyes that produce yellowish pus and mucus that may keep the eye from opening. A grating sensation or irritation in the eye or possibly burning or itching. The eyes may be sensitive to light. If left untreated, ulcers may form on the cornea of the eye, obscuring vision.

Areas to Treat/Types of Manipulation

Work both feet completely first. Then find locations of reflexes that correspond to these organs, and work them in the following order (see Chapter 3 for guidance):

1. Sinus/Head: Using thumb tip, first work tips of toes, using circular motion; then work all around the whole toe.
2. Eye/Ear: Apply direct circular pressure with thumb tip.
3. Kidneys: Apply direct pressure with thumb tip.
4. Adrenals: Apply direct pressure with thumb tip.

PREVENTIVE MEASURES AND COMPLEMENTARY TREATMENTS

Reflexology works well in conjunction with other alternative therapies and commonsense measures. For example:

WASH YOUR EYE: Gently remove excess mucus with a clean, warm washcloth. If you use the cloth again, use a different spot so that you don't reinfect yourself.

SHIELD YOUR EYES FROM LIGHT: Wear dark glasses or stay in dimly lit rooms while you're recuperating.

DON'T SHARE: Make sure you keep your handkerchiefs, towels, and washcloths to yourself; if only one eye is affected, use separate towels for each eye.

If commonsense hygiene and reflexology have not alleviated the symptoms within five days or if your eye is painful, consult your physician, who will prescribe antibiotic or steroid eyedrops to clear up the condition.

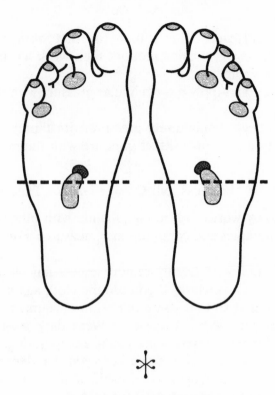

✳

CONSTIPATION

It's embarrassing, uncomfortable, and not the sort of thing you can discuss in public. Your belly puffs out in front of you; even though you try to alleviate the fullness, nothing moves.

Constipation is an inability to have regular bowel movements coupled with a lot of discomfort, gas, a distended abdomen, and often pain on defecation. Everyone has a different digestive system that takes less or more time to process nutrients and waste. If you are the type of person who has a very slow digestive system, and you regularly have a bowel movement every two to three days, but you have no other symptoms, you are not constipated. However, even if you manage to defecate daily but the bowels are hard and difficult to move, you are constipated.

Peristalsis moves food rhythmically from the gut to the intestines, and during the process of digestion, waste is separated out from the nutrients. The colon then removes water from the waste in order to form stools. Further waves of peristalsis move the stools out the rectum and anus. Any alterations in the amount of water removed or the speed of the muscular contractions can hamper the bowel. Several problems that might cause constipation can occur anywhere along this line.

The first problem may be the type of food you eat. A lot of fiber will help move other food along the digestive tract, and a lack of it may pose problems. Too much dairy food can cause constipation, as can a lack of food; if you're on a strict diet, you may have difficulty passing stools. A whole grain, fresh fruit, and vegetable diet will rid your body of toxins much faster than a red meat and fried food diet. Lots of fluids (8 to 10 glasses daily) can also help keep you regular.

The second problem is a use of laxatives. If you begin to rely on chemical laxatives to help you move your bowels, you may be unable to defecate without them.

Pregnancy can cause constipation. Because all the internal organs shift as the fetus grows, the bowel may be blocked or the additional weight of the fetus may keep the stool from passing easily. In addition, the increased hormone levels interfere with the intestinal muscle movements.

An intestinal blockage, colitis, or diverticulitis (the development of small extensions from the colon that can collect pockets of gas) may interfere with regular defecation.

A final problem is psychological. Many individuals get into a pattern of going to the bathroom at a certain time in a certain place. If they're traveling or for some reason they miss their special times of day and special places, they may feel that it's impossible to go. If the cycle continues, and they hold back for several days in a row, finally passing stools may be very difficult and painful. They may strain at their stools, damaging veins in the anus. The more blockage, the less water the bowels retain, and the harder the stool becomes. The fear of repeating this pain can set the cycle going again.

SYMPTOMS: A distended, uncomfortable, full feeling, accompanied by flatulence and the inability to pass stool. The act of trying may be painful and difficult. Very often gastrointestinal problems are further complicated by bad breath (caused by a buildup of toxins in the digestive tract), a coated tongue, and headaches.

Areas to Treat/Types of Manipulation

Work both feet completely first. Then find locations of reflexes that correspond to these organs, and work them in the following order (see Chapter 3 for guidance):

1. Colon: Beginning on the right foot, glide the thumb tip from the ileocecal valve up the ascending colon, across the transverse colon, to the inside edge of the foot.

   Continue with the left foot. Glide the thumb left to right across the transverse colon, down the descending colon, and end with a slight upward hook at the sigmoid colon.
2. Liver/Gallbladder: Apply direct pressure to the gallbladder reflex; then glide up and to the left across the liver reflex.
3. Adrenals: Apply direct pressure with thumb tip.

4. Solar Plexus: With the thumb tip, apply gradual pressure in the middle of the reflex, and work out to the edges.
5. Lower Back (Lumbar Spine): Glide the thumb tip down the inside of the foot from the base of the ball to the top of the heel.

PREVENTIVE MEASURES AND COMPLEMENTARY TREATMENTS

Reflexology works well in conjunction with other alternative therapies and commonsense measures. For example:

ADD FIBER TO YOUR DIET: By increasing the complex carbohydrates in your diet, you can start more activity in your gastrointestinal tract. Fruits and vegetables (with skins on) and whole grains provide a good amount of fiber. You should ideally get 30 grams daily. One bowl of bran cereal will provide 13 grams; half a cup of baked beans will give you 11 grams. Other good sources are prunes, figs, oatmeal, nuts, and popcorn.

EAT SOME PSYLLIUM: Psyllium seed (sold in health food stores) is a natural laxative. Try sprinkling it on food or eating Uncle Sam cereal, which contains this seed.

AVOID FOODS THAT MIGHT CONSTIPATE YOU: Rice and bananas are typically known as binding foods, and milk is also often a culprit in constipation. Gassy foods, such as broccoli, beans, and cabbage, may also be difficult for your system to process.

DRINK TO YOUR STOMACH'S CONTENT: The more fluids, the better. Remember that constipation is often due to water being removed from your food. So be sure to drink 8 to 10 eight-ounce glasses of pure springwater, fruit juice, or herbal tea every day.

RUN AROUND: Exercise is great for your bowel, as it is for all your body's organs. Walking, jogging, biking,

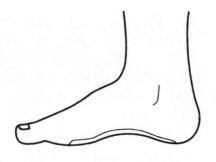

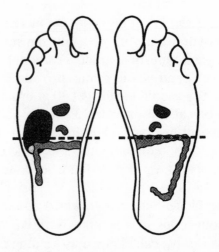

racquet sports, dance, and other aerobic activities help move the food through the bowel at a faster rate.

GET ON A REGULAR SCHEDULE: Set a regular time each day after a meal to sit on the toilet. Don't strain; just let it happen. You may be surprised to see that the regularity of simply being there can affect the process of your bowel.

If none of these measures provides relief, or if you have been constipated for more than three weeks, or if you have bloody stools, consult a physician.

COUGHS AND COLDS

The wheezes and sneezes are annoying; the tickle at the back of your throat makes it hard to swallow or talk. You're not feverish, but you just feel miserable. Did you catch this from someone on the train, or were you just so run-down it was your body's way of saying, "Take a rest"?

A cold, or upper respiratory infection, is the most common viral infection around. Cold viruses are often present in the air, but very often we don't pick them up unless our immune systems are compromised and can't combat the infectious cough or sneeze or contact with a germ-laden glass or spoon.

Colds usually don't last more than a week, and if they're mild, you can continue your work, but you sometimes feel so awful it's hard to get the energy to do much more than sleep or lie around watching TV. The danger of not pampering your cold symptoms is that by going about your business, you can exacerbate the symptoms and pick up a bacterial infection, such as bronchitis or sinusitis, at the same time.

You cannot catch a cold from going out without a coat in the winter, or from dancing in the rain, or from "catching a chill." If you already have cold symptoms, however, being cold and wet may increase them.

SYMPTOMS: Scratchy, tickling throat with frequent impetus to let out a dry cough. Sneezing and nasal discharge, fullness in the ears and sinuses, possible low-grade fever.

AREAS TO TREAT/TYPES OF MANIPULATION

Work both feet completely first. Then find locations of reflexes that correspond to these organs, and work them in the following order (see Chapter 3 for guidance):

1. Sinus/Head: Using the thumb tip, first work tips of toes, using circular motion; then work all around the whole toe.
2. Throat: Apply gradual direct pressure on reflex point. (CAUTION: This can be painful.)
3. Lungs: With tip and edge of thumb, work up and down and left to right.
4. Bronchi: With tip and edge of both thumbs, glide from the bases of the toes down toward the instep.
5. Spleen: Apply gradual circular pressure with thumb tip and pad.
6. Ileocecal Valve: Apply direct pressure with thumb tip.

PREVENTIVE MEASURES AND COMPLEMENTARY TREATMENTS

Reflexology works well in conjunction with other alternative therapies and commonsense measures. For example:

STOCK UP ON C: High doses of vitamin C may stave off a cold; it works better if you start supplementing as soon as you feel the first symptom. Take 500 mg. of C four times daily. (CAUTION: This may cause some gastrointestinal upset.)

DRINK SOMETHING HOT: The old panacea chicken soup works mainly because it's hot; the warmth gets the nasal passages flowing and clears the sinuses. If you get bored with soup, you can drink hot water with lemon juice or any of the herbal teas listed here.

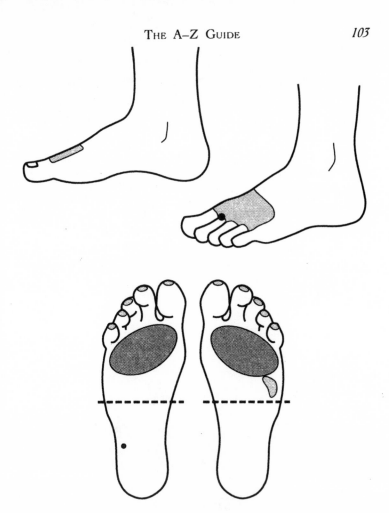

TRY SOME HERBS: Licorice root tea is excellent for colds, as is Traditional Medicinal's Throat Coat tea, which contains slippery elm bark, fennel seed, and orange peel in addition to licorice root. Avoid caffeineated teas that will make it more difficult for you to calm down and sleep.

GARGLE WITH SALT: Mix 1 teaspoon of salt in a glass of water, and gargle frequently. This will both break up the phlegm and soothe the throat.

SUCK ON SOMETHING: It's useful to keep the mucous

membranes of the throat lubricated, so keep cough drops or lozenges handy throughout the day and night.

GET SOME SLEEP: The body really wants to rest when it's fighting off a virus, so give it what it needs. Take a nap in the middle of the day, and turn in early at night.

BOOST YOUR IMMUNITY: Echinacea and goldenseal are a good herbal combination when you have a cold. Take half a dropperful of tincture three times daily.

If you have a fever over 103, or if you are producing yellow or greenish mucus when you cough, see your physician. Reflexology and other alternative treatments can help balance the immune system and spur recovery from your condition.

CYSTITIS

SEE URINARY TRACT INFECTIONS

DEPRESSION

You can't get out of bed in the morning. Nothing has any interest for you: not your job, your partner, your children. Even food and sex seem like too much trouble. Sometimes you get weepy for no reason; sometimes you're so angry you could throw plates. It's hard to concentrate when people talk to you, and you feel so tired you just want to crawl into a hole and seal yourself up in it.

Everyone feels "blue" occasionally, but if your feelings are ever-present no matter what is going on in your life or if your despondent reactions are out of proportion to the situation you're in, you may be clinically depressed. Depression can be a dangerous illness that affects one in four women and about half as many men. It may strike at any age, but typically it first appears in the mid to late twenties and then may vanish only to reappear at times of particular stress: after the birth of a baby, when taking a new job, at the death of a parent, or when entering midlife.

There are numerous possible causes for depression—physiological, psychological, spiritual, and environmental—but the manifestations are similar. The condition may be more prevalent in women partly because of hormonal fluctuation, but the many other factors include job status, learned helplessness, problems with interpersonal relationships, and overcommitment to many caregiver roles without allotting sufficient time for oneself. Depression can also be a reaction to such trauma as chronic pain, ongoing illness, childhood abuse, battering, or rape.

Depression can be partnered with eating and sleeping disorders, panic disorder, obsessive-compulsive disorder, and extreme mood swings. Bipolar disorder (which used to be called manic depression) involves periods of extremely "up" behavior—extravagant spending, creative bursts, wild socializing—with terribly "down" periods.

SYMPTOMS: Classic symptoms include a loss of interest in all activities; over- or undereating or sleeping; physical symptoms like headaches, stomachaches, or backaches that don't respond to any form of treatment; feelings of guilt and worthlessness; extreme fatigue; restlessness and irritability; abandoning personal hygiene; difficulty concentrating; and thoughts of suicide.

Areas to Treat/Types of Manipulation

Work both feet completely first. Then find the locations of reflexes that correspond to these organs, and work in the following order (see Chapter 3 for guidance):

1. Endocrine System (Adrenals, Ovaries or Testes, Thyroid/Parathyroid, Pituitary)

    Adrenals: Apply direct pressure with thumb tip.

    Ovaries/Testes: Apply gradual pressure with thumb tip and pad.

    Thyroid/Parathyroid: Work "necks" of toes with thumb tip.

    Pituitary: Apply direct pressure with thumb tip.

2. Solar Plexus: With thumb tip, apply gradual pressure in the middle of the reflex, and work out to the edges.

3. Pancreas: Apply direct circular pressure with thumb tip.

4. Head: Using thumb tip, first work tips of toes, using circular motion; then work all around the whole toe.

Preventive Measures and Complementary Treatments

Reflexology works well in conjunction with other alternative therapies and commonsense measures. For example:

CUT OUT SUGAR AND CAFFEINE: Sugar elevates blood glucose levels abruptly; then, as the effect wears off, levels drop precipitously. Caffeine stimulates the nervous system for about an hour but leaves you depressed and exhausted (and needing another cup of coffee). Try removing both from your diet, and see if you don't feel calmer.

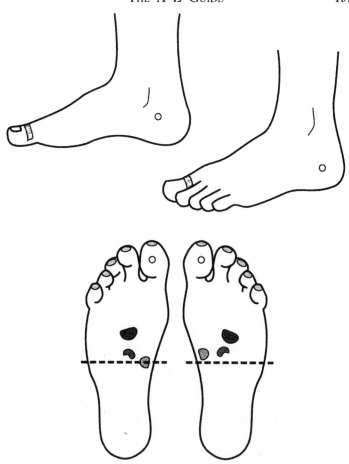

SUPPLEMENT YOUR DIET: Vitamin B complex, 50 mg. daily (particularly B$_6$, 100 mg. daily), is known as the "stress" vitamin, and it can make a big difference in your moods. Other helpful supplements for depression are the minerals calcium (1000–1200 mg. daily), magnesium (500–600 mg. daily), and zinc (30 mg daily).

TAKE AN HERB: Oat (*Avena sativa*), which nourishes the nervous system, has been touted as the great antidepressant of nature's kingdom. St.-John's-wort is excellent for treating moodiness and anxiety, although not for severe depression. Take 2 to 4 teaspoons dried herb infused in a cup of water or 30 drops of the tincture three times daily.

DRINK A FLOWER REMEDY: The Bach flower remedy for depression and hopelessness is gorse. For despondency and apathy, take gentian or wild rose. Mustard is for deep melancholy and gloom that descend without reason. Take 5 to 6 drops mixed in half a glass of water or directly under the tongue.

LISTEN TO MUSIC: It does have "charms to soothe a savage breast" and can really change your feelings. It's also a good idea to use music for your reflexology session every once in a while.

Select a particular type of music that moves you deeply: classical, jazz, Latin, Broadway musicals, or hip-hop. Then narrow your choice to a piece that is either upbeat or in some other way counter to the mood you're currently in. Take a twenty-minute break from whatever you're doing—no phone calls or conversations allowed—and sit quietly, letting the music wash over you. (Or work on your feet as you listen.)

Give yourself permission to get inside the rhythms and melodies, and let the music transform you. As the piece ends, be aware of the difference in your emotions, and try to keep that good feeling for the rest of the day. If you think you're losing it, call up the sound of the music in your mind, and get yourself back in the place you were in while listening.

GO OUT AND EXERCISE: Any type of activity that gets your heart rate up—jogging, biking, skating, dancing, racquet sports, etc.—begins the flow of beta-endorphins to the brain. These natural opiates, often responsible for the runner's high, provide us with a sense of well-being and can lift a depressed mood even hours after the exercise session is over.

HAVE A MASSAGE: Massage works in addition to and as an adjunct therapy to reflexology. The benefits are enormous, particularly the emotional boost from having someone touch you kindly and purposefully. Whether a professional or a friend is doing the massage, make sure he or she is aware that you need comforting and taking care of. This means no abrupt movements or uncomfortable pressure. When you are truly in someone else's hands, you have the opportunity to let go of your depression and allow the sensation of touch to heal you.

LEARN TO MEDITATE: Meditation is a time simply to be, to sit without any intention and observe the self you live with every day. It is also a time to clear the mind of worries, obsessions, and preoccupations. Take twenty minutes out of each day to sit quietly, either on a mat on the floor or in a straight-backed chair. Begin by observing your breath, watching it ebb and flow as it comes into you and moves out of you. If your mind wanders, bring it back to the breath. This constant rhythmic pattern that nourishes and supports you can be a helpmeet in a time of trouble. As you observe the life-giving force of the air and energy you absorb, you will discover other facets of you that are filled with life and hope.

TOUCH A PET: Many studies have proved that physical contact with a dog or cat lowers blood pressure and heart rate and can trigger the flow of neurotransmitters, the brain hormones that make us feel good. The unconditional love and close affection of a purring kitten or cuddly pup are a symbol of the life-affirming spirit that exists all around us if we only open our eyes to see it and allow it in. If you don't own an animal, you might want to experiment with a friend's pet; if you feel a good effect from the session, why not adopt a furry friend?

If five or more depressive symptoms persist for more than two weeks, it is crucial that you get professional help. Depression can kill, but it usually responds when treated early and aggressively, with psychotherapy and/ or mood-altering drugs. Reflexology and the alternative therapies listed above can alleviate some symptoms and make medical or psychological treatment proceed more smoothly.

DIABETES

There has never been a thirst like the one you're experiencing, and no amount of liquid seems to quench it. You are exhausted all the time; the other day you nearly passed out.

Diabetes mellitus is a malfunction of the endocrine system that makes it impossible for the body to metabolize and use sugar (glucose), the body's first fuel. The pancreas does not secrete enough of a hormone called insulin, whose job is to move the glucose from the bloodstream throughout the body into the various cells. What happens is that glucose begins to circulate freely and eventually spills into the urine since it is not used. The kidneys, which process the toxins and waste, are overloaded with excess sugar and in time may stop functioning. Diabetes can lead to kidney failure, cataracts and other eye problems, atherosclerosis, impotence, gangrene, and a lowered immune system. Women develop the disease more frequently than men; individuals who are obese have a greater predisposition to diabetes since the preponderance of fat cells leads to increased resistance to insulin.

There are two types of diabetes mellitus: Type 1 (insulin-dependent), common in children and young adults, results from a defect in a small part of the pancreas known as the islet of Langerhans. Type 2 (non–insulin-dependent), common in individuals over forty, may be triggered by a pancreas malfunction as well but is also caused by an insufficient number of insulin receptors on cells throughout the body. This means that insulin may be present in the body but can't be used. Another trigger of late-onset diabetes is pregnancy. This typically occurs in women who carry babies that weigh more than ten pounds at birth.

SYMPTOMS: *Type 1:* excessive thirst and urination, fatigue, vision problems, dizziness and fainting, increased appetite, high concentration of sugar apparent in urine test, weight loss.

Type 2: Sometimes none; sometimes same as above. However, it is more typical that the individual does not lose weight. Also, slow and difficult healing of injuries and cuts.

AREAS TO TREAT/TYPES OF MANIPULATION

Work both feet completely first. Then find the locations of reflexes that correspond to these organs, and work in the following order (see Chapter 3 for guidance):

1. Pancreas: Apply direct circular pressure with thumb tip.
2. Pituitary: Apply direct pressure with thumb tip.
3. Thyroid: Work "necks" of toes with thumb tip.
4. Liver/gallbladder: Apply direct pressure to gallbladder; then glide up and to left across liver.
5. Adrenals: Apply direct pressure with thumb tip.

PREVENTIVE MEASURES AND COMPLEMENTARY TREATMENTS

Reflexology works well in conjunction with other alternative therapies and commonsense measures. For example:

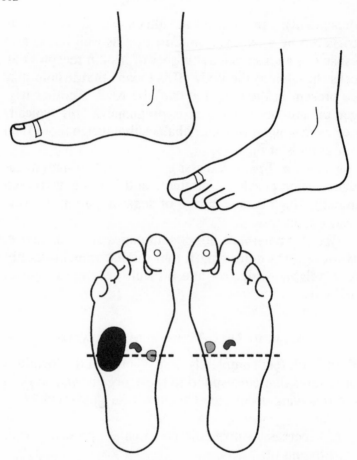

EAT RIGHT: The American Diabetes Association provides excellent guidelines for eating, including a diet
that is 50 to 60 percent carbohydrates, 12 to 20 percent
protein, and 20 to 30 percent fat. Your physician will
undoubtedly recommend that you see a dietitian to cus-
tom-design a program of healthy eating. If blood sugar
is too high (hyperglycemia), you may experience weakness, fatigue, and thirst; if it drops too low (hypoglycemia), you may be ravenously hungry, start to sweat and
tremble, develop a headache, feel as if your mouth is

numb, become dizzy, and possibly pass out. For this reason, eat smaller meals more often so that the sugar and carbohydrates you consume (which metabolize into sugar in the body) will keep your blood glucose concentration on an even keel.

GO HEAVY ON FIBER: Fiber lowers cholesterol, which lowers the amount of fat in your blood. It also allows sugar to be absorbed more slowly, and that keeps glucose levels pretty stable. Try eating about 25 to 40 grams of vegetables, fruits (with skin), whole wheat products, barley, oats, and legumes daily.

SHED SOME POUNDS IF YOU ARE OVERWEIGHT: Work with your doctor and dietitian so that you can lose slowly and steadily until you are within the weight range for your height recommended by life insurance tables.

GET OUT AND EXERCISE: Establishing a program of walking, swimming, biking, dance, or low-impact aerobics (about a half hour daily) will make you feel like sticking with your diet and will also provide a boost of needed energy so essential to a diabetic. Exercise also strengthens the heart and circulatory system and helps control blood sugar levels. There is also some evidence that it increases the number of insulin receptors on cell surfaces.

Diabetes is a serious condition and must be under the close supervision of a physician. Reflexology and the alternative therapies listed above can strengthen the endocrine system and make insulin, when injected, more readily available to the tissues.

DIVERTICULITIS

That sharp, stabbing pain on the left side! What could it be? At the same time you feel sick to your stomach and slightly feverish. Your elimination system hasn't been normal lately: Sometimes you have diarrhea; sometimes you're constipated.

The problem is an inflammation of the diverticula, little grapelike pouches that form when the inner lining of the colon is forced through weak spots in the outer layer because it's under too much pressure. This pressure occurs when there is too little bulk (fiber) to create adequate movement through the large intestine.

Most Westerners eat a diet low in fiber and high in processed foods. More than half of all Americans over sixty have diverticulosis, the chronic form of this problem, when pouches form along the outer wall of the colon. Diverticulosis usually has no symptoms. The acute form, diverticulitis, occurs when a mass of hardened waste forms in one of these pouches and presses against the outer wall, where they may be infected by the bacteria that live in the colon. This inflamed section may rupture or attach itself to another organ—usually the bladder or vagina—creating a fistula, or an abnormal passageway that leaks infectious material. The more frequently the inflammations develop, the more likely it is for the colon to thicken and narrow, causing a partial or total obstruction of the bowel.

SYMPTOMS: Acute or cramplike pain in the lower left quadrant of the abdomen, or occasionally in other areas of the abdomen, sometimes accompanied by nausea and fever. Possible pain on urination, constipation or diarrhea, or both.

AREAS TO TREAT/TYPES OF MANIPULATION

Work both feet completely first. Then find the locations of reflexes that correspond to these organs, and work in the following order (see Chapter 3 for guidance):

1. Colon: Beginning on the right foot, apply direct pressure with thumb tip to the ileocecal valve; then glide the thumb tip from this valve up the ascending colon, across the transverse colon, to the inside edge of the foot.

   Switch to the left foot. Glide the thumb tip left to right across the transverse colon, down the descending colon, and end with a slight hook upward at the sigmoid colon.
2. Sigmoid Colon: Apply direct pressure with thumb tip.
3. Solar Plexus: With thumb tip, apply gradual pressure in the middle of the reflex, and work out to the edges.
4. Adrenals: Apply direct pressure with thumb tip.

PREVENTIVE MEASURES AND COMPLEMENTARY TREATMENTS

Reflexology works well in conjunction with other alternative therapies and commonsense measures. For example:

EAT YOUR FIBER: In addition to high-fiber foods, such as fruits (with skin), vegetables, whole grain products, legumes, barley, and bran, you can take psyllium, a supplement found in natural laxatives such as Metamucil. If you are currently not a big fiber eater, you should increase amounts slowly, at the same time cutting down

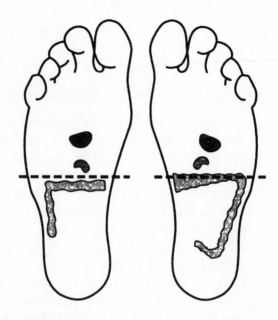

on processed foods, so as not to shock your gastrointestinal system.

CUT OUT SEEDS AND NUTS: These small, hard foods are difficult to digest and may become lodged in the diverticula, causing pain. It's best to eliminate these items from your diet if you know that you have diverticulosis or diverticulitis.

DON'T CONSUME BOWEL IRRITANTS: Caffeine and alcohol can irritate the bowel. You might try to reduce or eliminate both and see whether your system likes the change.

DRINK LIQUIDS: Be sure you drink 8 to 10 glasses of liquid (pure springwater, herbal teas, and juices) each day to break down the food as it passes through your system.

TAKE A STOOL SOFTENER: In order to avoid the deposit of hard waste, you can take a stool softener daily. These are available in drugstores.

GET ACTIVE: Exercise allows freer passage of digested materials and makes defecation easier, with no strain.

If reflexology and appropriate dietary changes do not alleviate your symptoms, you should consult a physician who will do a full examination and possibly a barium X ray to locate diverticula and fistulas and to rule out cancer of the colon.

Dizziness (Vertigo)

It comes on without warning and nearly knocks you over. You feel the world spinning and see spots before your eyes. Suddenly you feel sick to your stomach, your hands turn clammy, your face turns pale.

Vertigo, or dizziness, is a symptom of something that affects control centers in the brain stem or balance in the middle ear. It might occur because you have a high fever, because you've consumed too much alcohol or have a reaction to medication, because you have a mild concussion, or because you got up too fast (orthostatic hypotension). It is also a symptom of multiple sclerosis, brain cancer, and Ménière's disease, a condition of the middle ear that may eventually bring on deafness.

Some individuals are better able to tolerate vertigo than others. One of the criteria for becoming a test pilot or astronaut, for example, is being able to withstand many times the pull of gravity and violent spinning in centrifugelike machines. People with exceptionally developed middle ears may experience only mild discomfort, whereas many of us find even an amusement park ride sick-making.

SYMPTOMS: A sense that everything is moving around you or that your brain is moving within your skull. In addition, you may have clammy hands and nausea, and your face may suddenly turn white.

Areas to Treat/Types of Manipulation

Work both feet completely first. Then find the locations of the eye and ear reflexes, and work them carefully (see Chapter 3 for guidance):

Eye/Ear: Apply direct circular pressure with thumb tip.

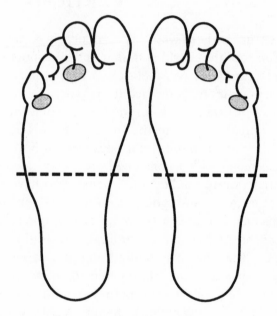

Preventive Measures and Complementary Treatments

Reflexology works well in conjunction with other alternative therapies and commonsense measures. For example:

GET UP SLOWLY: If you tend to feel dizzy, particularly after meals, when you go from a seated to a standing position, take plenty of time to complete the move. If you get up in the middle of the night, turn on your side, and dangle your feet off the edge of the bed before coming to a standing position.

GET OFF ALCOHOL AND DRUGS: Remember before you overindulge how awful it makes you feel, and then refrain! If you're on an over-the-counter or prescription medication that makes you woozy, don't drink or operate heavy machinery. Consult your physician about changing medications or lowering the dosage of the one you're on.

FOCUS ON YOURSELF: When the world is spinning, try looking directly at a part of your own body—your arm or hand. Just the act of focusing your attention on one object will make the range of perceived movement around you smaller and easier to handle.

If reflexology and the commonsense therapies have not alleviated your dizziness, or if you become dizzy more frequently than you used to, consult a physician for a full workup to rule out any serious illnesses.

EARACHES

There's a red-hot throbbing pain in your ear—sometimes a dull ache, but more often a searing inflammation that makes you feel feverish and miserable. Sometimes your ears pop; sometimes you just can't hear a thing.

An earache may stem from several different causes: an outer, an inner, or, most commonly, a middle ear infection (otitis media), or mastoiditis (a bacterial infection of the mastoid air cells behind the ear that is often a complication of a middle ear infection). Water in the ear after swimming or airplane travel may give you pain in your ears. Teething (in infants), severe tooth decay, or a sinus infection may also cause one or both ears to ache.

Infections in the ear occur when a virus or bacterium in the nose or throat passes through the eustachian tube, which connects these organs to the middle ear. If the infection is serious or occurs often (as it does in many young children), it may actually cause the eardrum to bulge and burst, causing pus to leak into the external ear canal. Earaches tend to be worse at night when you lie down and the eustachian tubes can't drain properly, as they do when you're standing or sitting up.

SYMPTOMS: An ache or pain in the ear, high fever (sometimes it will elevate to 102 degrees in adults and 105 degrees in children), dizziness, hearing loss, loss of appetite, nausea, vomiting, sore throat, loss of balance. You may have some pus or blood-tinged pus emanating from the ear.

AREAS TO TREAT/TYPES OF MANIPULATION

Work both feet completely first. Then find the locations of the eye and ear reflexes, and work them carefully (see Chapter 3 for guidance):

Eye/Ear: Apply direct circular pressure with thumb tip.

PREVENTIVE MEASURES AND COMPLEMENTARY TREATMENTS

Reflexology works well in conjunction with other alternative therapies and commonsense measures. For example:

CHANGE POSITION AND SWALLOW: Sometimes tilting your

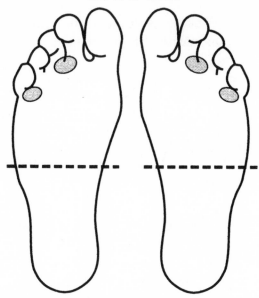

head a different way can make the pain subside. Swallowing gets air into the middle ear, preventing a painful vacuum. Be sure to sleep propped up on lots of pillows.

CHEW GUM; DRINK LIQUIDS: The muscular action of chewing and swallowing will open your ears and alleviate the ache.

USE WARMTH: A heating pad or a warm hot-water bottle wrapped in a towel, held against the ear, may make it feel better.

DON'T PUT ANYTHING IN THE EAR: Ear swabs (to remove wax) are not recommended when your eardrum is bulging. Also, don't use commercial preparations or warm mineral oil unless you've okayed them with your doctor.

STAY AWAY FROM SMOKE: Cigarette smoke, wood smoke from a fire, and air pollution will adversely affect your ears, nose, and throat (which are all connected).

You should consult a physician about any earache that does not respond to reflexology or alternative treatments within three days. He or she will prescribe an antibiotic and analgesics to treat the problem. Prolonged infection may lead to permanent hearing loss.

Eczema (see also Skin Disorders, p. 264)

It is too embarrassing. Those red, swollen, oozing blisters that look like something out of a science fiction movie; the scaling, crusting, and scabbing over that take place afterward. You know it's just a severe form of dermatitis (inflammation of the skin), but you can't imagine that other people can stand to look at you.

Eczema, also known as atopic dermatitis, is a severe form of skin inflammation that often affects the flexor muscles, such as the elbow or knee. Some forms of the condition are caused by food allergies (usually to wheat, eggs, or milk) as well as by inhalant allergens and sensitivity to ragweed pollen, which can lead to other problems, such as hay fever or asthma, but other forms of eczema have no relation whatsoever to allergies. Some dermatologists believe the cause is heredity; others think that emotional factors can trigger outbreaks of the rash.

There is no cure for eczema. However, good preventive health measures such as reflexology and other complementary treatments can ease the discomfort and minimize the unappealing look of the condition.

SYMPTOMS: Variable, from red, blistering rash with oozing blisters to low-grade thickening and discoloration of the skin. The intense itching that occurs is usually triggered by changing clothes, touching wool or animal fur, or sweating. Scratching the eczema thickens the skin, and thickened skin tends to itch more.

Many people with eczema have particularly dry skin and may have bumpy rashes on the thighs and upper arms. They are also more prone to boils and other skin infections.

AREAS TO TREAT/TYPES OF MANIPULATION

Work both feet completely first. Then find the locations of reflexes that correspond to these organs, and work in the following order (see Chapter 3 for guidance):

1. Endocrine System (Adrenals, Ovaries or Testes, Thyroid/Parathyroid, Pituitary)
   Adrenals: Apply direct pressure with thumb tip.
   Ovaries/Testes: Apply gradual pressure with thumb tip and pad.
   Thyroid/Parathyroid: Work "necks" of toes with thumb tip.
   Pituitary: Apply direct pressure with thumb tip.
2. Solar Plexus: With thumb tip, apply gradual pressure in the middle of the reflex, and work out to the edges
3. Kidneys: Apply direct pressure with thumb tip.
4. Lymph Glands: Work thumb tip and pad gently back and forth across area.

PREVENTIVE MEASURES AND COMPLEMENTARY TREATMENTS

Reflexology works well in conjunction with other alternative therapies and commonsense measures. For example:

KEEP YOUR SKIN MOIST: To avoid the itching of dry skin (which will make you scratch more), apply a

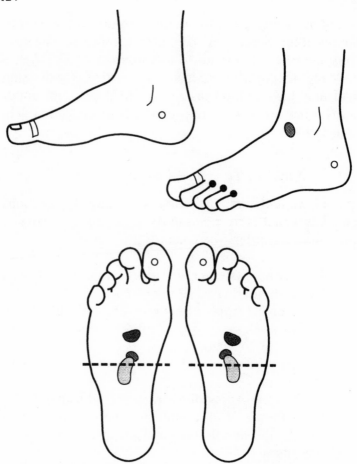

nonperfumed lubricating lanolin-based lotion or cream several times a day.

STAY CLEAR OF ITCHY FIBERS: Don't allow your body to touch wool, animal fur, synthetics, or drying soaps. Dress in loose clothing made of cotton or silk.

BE AWARE OF ALLERGIC FOOD REACTIONS: Keep a food diary, and note when your outbreaks occur. If you see that you've consumed a particular food (particularly one that commonly causes allergic reactions), stay away from it.

DON'T SCRATCH: Meditation and visualization can often help you "convince" yourself that your skin doesn't itch. Imagine that you are covered with a smooth, impenetrable shield that bonds to your skin and makes it completely comfortable. Shift your area of focus from the patch that itches to one that doesn't, and you may find that the two meld in your mind. If you can control your first impulse to scratch, the desire will eventually fade.

If reflexology and the other alternative treatments listed above have not alleviated the itching and unsightly condition of your eczema, consult a physician who will prescribe an antibiotic cream and/or a steroid preparation to treat the condition.

EDEMA

You feel bloated, and your body seems to be all puffed up like a balloon. When you press on your leg, the sensation is like depressing a piece of clay with your thumb: The skin doesn't bounce back; it's lost all elasticity.

Edema is retention of excess fluid, and it may occur in one area or all over the body. Water retention may be caused by exceptionally serious conditions, such as kidney disorders, congestive heart failure, cirrhosis of the liver, or a concussion that causes fluid buildup in the brain. Or it may be caused by the monthly occurrence of hormonal fluctuation; edema is a common partner of PMS, pregnancy, and oral contraceptives. A lack of vitamin B can also make you swell up, as can a job that keeps you on your feet all the time.

The reason the body retains water is an imbalance

between the amount of fluid in the cells pumped by the capillaries and the amount taken back into them after nutrients and other chemicals have been delivered to the cells. In kidney disease the kidneys aren't able to excrete their requisite amount of fluid, which backs up in the bloodstream and is then displaced in the tissues. In heart disease blood stagnates in the veins and prevents the reabsorption of water from the tissues.

SYMPTOMS: Bloating, retention of urine, swelling of various body parts. If you have pitting edema, typical of congestive heart failure, you can create "pits" in the skin by pressing various places; the area will remain depressed after you let go.

AREAS TO TREAT/TYPES OF MANIPULATION

Work both feet completely first. Then find the locations of reflexes that correspond to these organs, and work in the following order (see Chapter 3 for guidance):

1. Kidneys: Apply direct pressure with thumb tip.
2. Adrenals: Apply direct pressure with thumb tip.

PREVENTIVE MEASURES AND COMPLEMENTARY TREATMENTS

Reflexology works well in conjunction with other alternative therapies and commonsense measures. For example:

GET OFF YOUR FEET: Putting your feet up will reduce the swelling in your ankles. If you have to stand for most of the day, get yourself good support stockings.

CUT OUT SALT: Salt in the diet makes the tissues retain fluid. This means you should eliminate or cut out salt, depending on your doctor's recommendation, and use other seasonings to flavor your food.

DON'T DRINK TOO MUCH: If you are on dialysis, *you must*

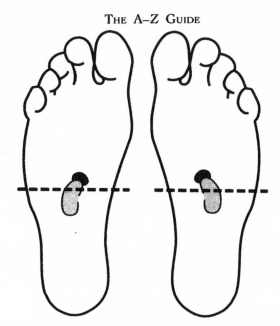

restrict your intake of fluids drastically. This is also true of other conditions, such as heart disease, in which diuretics will be prescribed to get more fluid out of the body.

You must be under a doctor's care for any condition other than normal hormonal fluctuations that cause fluid retention. Reflexology and alternative treatments will help restore fluid balance so that the body can respond more effectively to medication.

EMPHYSEMA

You can't breathe. You fill your lungs, but your chest doesn't even expand. You are exhausted with the effort of just having a conversation or moving from chair to couch.

Emphysema is a serious and debilitating lung disease caused by the loss of elasticity in the alveoli (air sacs) and bronchi (bronchial tubes that lead from the trachea to the lungs). The sacs and tubes become permanently distended with air as the patient tries unsuccessfully to get more oxygen, and a great deal of mucus develops in the lungs. At the same time the number of blood vessels in the lungs declines, and the amount of oxygen carried in the blood is reduced even further.

As the lungs become more like blown-out balloons that can't bounce back, it becomes more difficult for them to take in sufficient oxygen on the inhalation and to eliminate carbon dioxide with the exhalation. The lungs may actually collapse and require immediate surgery to restore at least partial function.

Emphysema also affects the heart and cardiovascular system. As the disease worsens, the heart has to pump much harder to get blood through the lungs, and it must pump a greater volume of blood for any exertion; even turning over in bed or standing up can require a major effort. Over time this strain on the heart may cause congestive heart failure.

This disease is most common in men over forty. It can cause the patient to become housebound and dependent on an oxygen tank, and it invariably leads to death.

The leading cause of emphysema is smoking, but people with chronic bronchitis also develop it, as do those exposed to continuous high levels of dust or pollution.

SYMPTOMS: Breathlessness and a heavy cough that can be brought on by talking or laughing. The condition is particularly uncomfortable after eating, when the lungs are expanded and the diaphragm drops down toward the stomach. For this reason, many emphysema sufferers don't eat properly or in the proper amount and become thin and wasted.

Many patients develop expanded barrel chests and a blue coloration in the skin, lips, and fingernails, the result of a lack of oxygen in the tissues.

AREAS TO TREAT/TYPES OF MANIPULATION

Work both feet completely first. Then find the locations of reflexes that correspond to these organs, and work in the following order (see Chapter 3 for guidance):

1. Bronchi: With the tip and edge of thumbs, glide from the base of the toes down toward the instep.
2. Lungs: With the tip and edge of thumb, work up and down and left to right.
3. Solar Plexus: With the thumb tip, apply gradual pressure in the middle of the reflex, and work out to edges.
4. Ileocecal Valve: Apply direct pressure with thumb tip.
5. Colon: Beginning on the right foot, glide the thumb tip from the ileocecal valve up the ascending colon, across the transverse colon, to the inside edge of the foot.
   Continue with the left foot. Glide the thumb left to right across the transverse colon, down the descending colon, and end with a slight upward hook.
6. Small Intestine: Glide the thumb back and forth and up and down throughout this reflex area.
7. Kidney/Adrenals: Apply direct pressure with thumb tip.

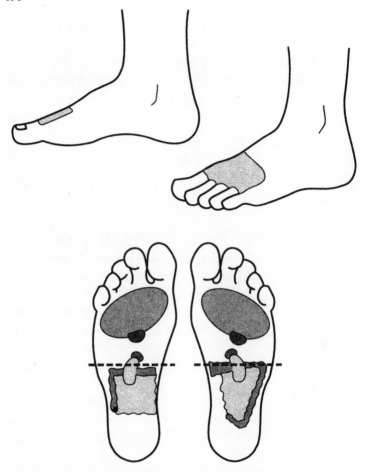

Preventive Measures and Complementary Treatments

Reflexology works well in conjunction with other alternative therapies and commonsense measures. For example:

COOL THE AIR: Use dehumidifiers and air conditioners to moisturize and filter the air you breathe.

AVOID IRRITANTS: Make sure you stay clear of paint fumes, automobile exhausts, strong perfumes, and cooking odors.

COVER YOUR MOUTH: Cold air can start up a spasm in your bronchial passages, so if it's bitter outside, keep a scarf or mask over your mouth and nose.

DRINK FLUIDS: Consuming at least eight 8-ounce glasses of pure water, fruit juice, and herbal tea will help thin out the mucus in your lungs and make it easier to breathe.

GET OUT AND WALK: Moderate exercise—walking or slow bicycling—is excellent to increase your tolerance for increased respiration. Start slowly, and do a little every day.

BREATHE RIGHT: Learn some directed breathing techniques that will strengthen the muscles in charge of inhalation and exhalation.

- *Belly Breathing:* This exercise gives your lungs a rest. Try not to let your chest expand when you use your belly. Lie on the floor, and place your hand on your abdomen. As you inhale, push your hand in, and as you exhale, resist as you press the hand out again.
- *Pursed Lip Breathing:* Using the belly breathing above, purse your lips and let the air out in a steady stream as though you were whistling. Take the air in again through open lips to give a wider passage for the inhalation.
- *Forced Breathing:* Inhale quickly, thrusting your shoulders back and exhale, forcing air out again. (Do only three of these in a session, and if you feel light-headed, stop at once.)

You must be under a doctor's care if you have emphysema. Reflexology and other alternative therapies should provide additional relief to your medication and oxygen replacement.

EYE PAIN

Someone has stuck something in your eye, under your lid, and the tearing just won't stop. Your eye is red and swollen and leaks a type of yellow pus. Or else you can see dry crusts along the surface of the lid, and normal daylight seems like a blinding floodlight.

Various conditions may cause pain in the eye, ranging from a simple sty or conjunctivitis to toxic amblyopia (usually a complication of chronic alcoholism) and acute glaucoma.

SYMPTOMS: *A Sty:* A sty is an inflamed or infected sebaceous gland in the eye. This oil-producing gland may be attacked by a bacterium that causes a painful lump on the eyelid. Once the sty bursts, and the fluid is released, the pain usually ceases.

Conjunctivitis: Also called pinkeye, this condition is caused by an inflammation of the conjunctiva, the lining of the eyelid and surface of the eye. It may cause redness, a gritty feeling in the eye, burning, itching, and light sensitivity.

Toxic Amblyopia: This condition is almost exclusively found in heavy drinkers and smokers as well as individuals exposed to toxic chemicals in the workplace. The toxic substances cause swelling of the optic nerve, resulting in pain whenever the eyeball moves in its socket. Poor eyesight and even blindness may result from this condition if left untreated.

Acute Glaucoma: This very rare condition may bring on pain in the eye so severe that it causes an upset of the entire system, including such symptoms as nausea and vomiting. It will also cause abrupt blurring of vision.

THIS IS AN EXCEPTIONALLY SERIOUS CONDITION, AND IMMEDI-
ATE MEDICAL CARE IS REQUIRED TO PREVENT BLINDNESS.

AREAS TO TREAT/TYPES OF MANIPULATION

Work both feet completely first. Then find the locations
of reflexes that correspond to these organs, and work in
the following order (see Chapter 3 for guidance):

1. Sinus/Head: Using thumb tip, first work the tips of
   the toes using circular motion; then work all
   around the whole toe.
2. Eye/Ear: Apply direct circular pressure with thumb
   tip.
3. Neck: Using thumb and index finger, manipulate
   "necks" of toes thoroughly.
4. Kidneys: Apply direct pressure with thumb tip.

PREVENTIVE MEASURES AND COMPLEMENTARY TREATMENTS

Reflexology works well in conjunction with other alternative therapies and commonsense measures. For example:

SHIELD YOUR EYES, BUT DON'T TOUCH: Wear dark glasses
to protect your eyes from glare. This will also help re-
mind you not to touch the painful eye (which might
introduce bacteria into it).

KEEP THE EYE CLEAN: If the eye is runny, be sure to
clean it every few hours with a moist sterile gauze pad.
Always turn the pad after one swipe so as to get a clean
surface for the next swipe. Always use a fresh pad to
clean the second eye.

DON'T USE COMMERCIAL EYEDROPS: Eyedrops that
"soothe" the eyes or "get the red out" may contain
chemicals that may irritate the eye further.

DON'T TREAT YOURSELF WITH OLD EYEDROPS: If you've

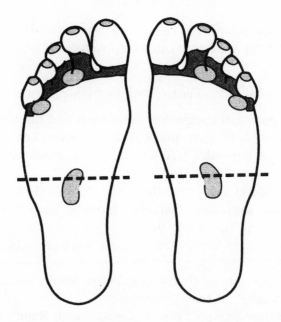

had recurrent eye infections or conditions that cause pain, you should use a fresh prescription each time. Discard whatever medication you haven't used at the end of the course of treatment.

It's a good idea to consult an ophthalmologist if you are having pain in your eye. Reflexology and other alternative treatments can remove blockages in the area so that medication will work more quickly and effectively.

Fatigue

You're as tired when you awake in the morning as when you go to sleep at night; your body feels as if a weight of bricks covered every inch of it. Nothing feels right or exciting, as though you'd lost the will to enjoy life. The only appealing thought is going to bed and sleeping for a year.

Fatigue is different from exhaustion, which is the body's natural reaction to working really hard and depleting its resources. It's not as simple to recover from a malady like fatigue that seems to have no cause and doesn't get better with rest.

Fatigue may be physical or emotional or both. You may be completely worn out from a stressful existence, or you may be run-down from a poor diet and bad sleep habits. Or you may also be depressed (see Depression, p. 104), a state that drains you of energy. Typical physical problems that might cause fatigue are illness, a low-grade infection, a lack of appropriate nutrients, an accumulation of waste products in the body, or an adrenal imbalance. Typical emotional problems that could bring it on are low self-esteem and lack of motivation. A more general problem, very common in women, is the fatigue brought on by juggling too many responsibilities at once—home, job, children, elderly parents, volunteer work, etc.

Fatigue is common at certain times of life: During adolescence, as children go through a growth spurt, they often sleep away entire weekends. Pregnancy is equally demanding since you're supporting another human being inside you. Menopause (and midlife change for men) can also bring with it periods of extreme fatigue, as hormonal imbalances sap you of your normal strengths. Advanced old age is a time when fatigue is likely to strike, though it is by no means the case that all elderly individuals have to feel fatigued.

Fatigue can be a symptom of a more serious illness. Anemia, chronic fatigue syndrome, diabetes, and lung disease all can make you feel washed out and weak as a kitten.

SYMPTOMS: A leaden, heavy feeling in body and mind. Inability to motivate yourself to get through daily chores, let alone begin new projects. A feeling of weakness and persistent tiredness, as if it's too much effort to hold your head up. Possibly also shortness of breath with any activity, even walking to the mailbox and back.

AREAS TO TREAT/TYPES OF MANIPULATION

Work both feet completely first. Then find the locations of reflexes that correspond to these organs, and work in the following order (see Chapter 3 for guidance):

1. Endocrine Glands (Adrenals, Ovaries or Testes, Thyroid/Parathyroid, Pituitary)
   Adrenals: Apply direct pressure with thumb tip.
   Ovaries or Testes: Apply gradual circular pressure with thumb tip and pad.
   Thyroid/Parathyroid: Work "necks" of toes with thumb tip.
   Pituitary: Apply direct pressure with thumb tip.
2. Solar Plexus: With thumb tip, apply gradual pressure in the center of the reflex and work out to the edges.
3. Adrenals: Apply direct pressure with thumb tip.
4. Colon: Beginning on the right foot, glide the thumb tip from the ileocecal valve up the ascending colon, across the transverse colon, to the inside edge of the foot.
   Continue with the left foot. Glide the thumb left to right across the transverse colon, down the descending colon, and end with a slight upward hook at the sigmoid colon.

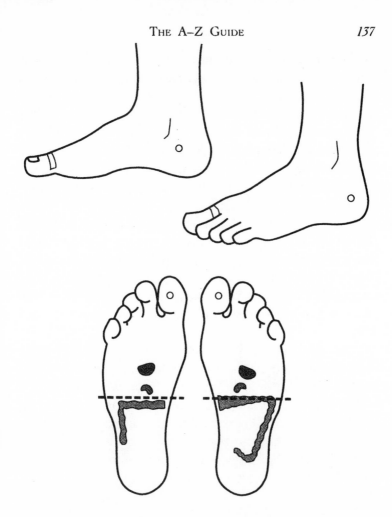

PREVENTIVE MEASURES AND COMPLEMENTARY TREATMENTS

Reflexology works well in conjunction with other alternative therapies and commonsense measures. For example:

GET ON A REGULAR SCHEDULE: Be sure you get at least seven hours' sleep at night, and don't nap during the day. Keep the same schedule on weekends as weekdays.

MOVE AROUND!: When you're most tired, that's when you should go out and exercise. A brisk two-mile walk or bike ride; a few laps in the pool; a low-impact aerobics, dance, or martial arts class will trigger the production in the brain of beta-endorphins, those neurotransmitters that act as natural opiates and fill us with a sense of well-being.

EAT RIGHT: Eliminate junk food and foods high in fats. Concentrate on whole grains, fresh fruits and vegetables, and drink 8 to 10 glasses of liquid (springwater, juice, or herbal tea) daily.

CAN THE CAFFEINE: Most people use coffee and caffeinated sodas as pick-me-ups when they feel they need an energy boost. Actually the chemicals in these products initially stimulate the brain and then, about an hour later, send you spiraling back down farther than you were before. Get off caffeine to get more energy in your day.

TURN OFF THE TUBE: The television set induces a sense of lethargy and has an almost hypnotic effect on the mind. This further dulls your senses when what you really want to do is enliven them. Instead of tuning in, turn on a great CD and read a book or magazine. Or go out with friends for a boost.

If neither reflexology nor any of the alternative therapies listed above alleviate your fatigue, consult your physician.

FEVER

It comes on suddenly—that haze that starts to close your eyes and make your muscles feel as though they can't support your bones. You just want to lie down and sleep and do so for hours, until you are awakened by violent chills that make your teeth chatter. The idea of eating is repellent, and your head pounds whenever you try to lift it off the pillow.

A fever is the body's reaction to an infection; in fact, if it is short-lived, it is a positive sign that the body is healing itself. When a foreign invader such as bacteria or a virus enters the body, the immune system starts fighting back in numerous ways. Fever is a first-line defense, triggered by the hypothalamus, the master gland in the brain that regulates temperature. A fever kills off those microorganisms that can't survive at higher temperatures. At the same time the immune system produces a variety of natural killer cells and other white blood cells that fight the invader.

Fever can't last too long. The body would be harmed if these elevated temperatures persisted, too much moisture would be absorbed, and the various organs would eventually "fry" at an elevated heat level. So the hypothalamus, ever a good manager of checks and balances, quickly drops the external temperature, producing violent chills. As the infection dies down, and this powerful defense mechanism is no longer necessary, the body temperature returns to normal.

AREAS TO TREAT/TYPES OF MANIPULATION

Work both feet completely first. Then find the location of the pituitary reflex, and work it carefully (see Chapter 3 for guidance):

Pituitary: Apply direct pressure with thumb tip.

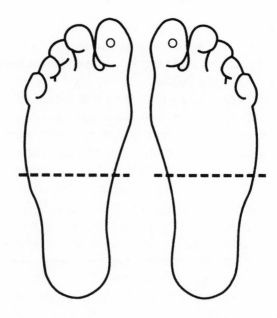

Preventive Measures and Complementary Treatments

Reflexology works well in conjunction with other alternative therapies and commonsense measures. For example:

GO TO BED: Don't try to carry on with your regular chores; you'll only make yourself sicker and possibly infect other people. Just take the time off and give in to the fever for a few days.

DRINK PLENTY OF LIQUIDS: When you have a fever and sweat a lot, you can become dehydrated. Since solid food won't seem palatable anyway, this is the time to consume plenty of fruit and vegetable juices; herb teas, such as black elder, linden, and willow bark; and pure springwater. You may suck on ice chips if you don't think you can keep anything down.

TAKE A SPONGE BATH: The old remedy for fevers, an alcohol bath, is not a good idea since alcohol will dry the body more than it already is and the patient may inhale the vapors or absorb them through the skin. Instead use plain cool tap water, and sponge off your head and neck, chest, armpits, and groin. Be sure to dry off with a towel so you don't get a chill afterward.

TRY SOME ASPIRIN: You may take aspirin every four hours as long as your physician allows it. Children with fever should always take Tylenol, however, since aspirin can trigger a serious neurological disease known as Reye's syndrome.

If neither reflexology nor any of the alternative therapies listed above bring down your fever within five days, or if your fever is accompanied by a stiff neck, or if your child of under four months has a high fever, consult your physician.

FLATULENCE

Oops. There you go again. It sounds bad, it smells worse, and there's nothing you can do to stop it. Passing gas is uncomfortable (until it's over) and terribly embarrassing. People move away from you as though you'd done something really gross.

Flatulence is natural; there are cultures where, like belching, passing gas is not considered impolite. However, if you commonly pass gas, there may be something wrong with your digestion.

When the stomach and intestines become distended with gas, this is sometimes because you have inhaled too much air while swallowing food or drink. When the air passes into the intestine, it meets up with the gas that naturally forms as bacteria work on the food you've consumed. Too much extra gas simply has to go somewhere. You generally get rid of some of it by belching or burping; the rest comes out the other end. This problem may also occur because you have an abundance of bacterial activity going on in your digestive tract.

Flatulence is generally just an annoyance. However, if accompanied by cramps and abdominal pain, it may be a symptom of irritable bowel, Crohn's disease, an ulcer, or a hiatal hernia.

SYMPTOMS: Air escaping forcibly from the anus; a "whoopie cushion" sound; a sulfurous odor similar to that of rotten eggs.

AREAS TO TREAT/TYPES OF MANIPULATION

Work both feet completely first. Then find the locations of reflexes that correspond to these organs, and work in the following order (see Chapter 3 for guidance):

1. Sigmoid Colon: Apply direct pressure with thumb tip.
2. Solar Plexus: With thumb tip, apply gradual pressure in the center of the reflex, and work out to the edges.
3. Small Intestine: Glide thumb back and forth and up and down through area.

PREVENTIVE MEASURES AND COMPLEMENTARY TREATMENTS

Reflexology works well in conjunction with other alternative therapies and commonsense measures. For example:

CHANGE YOUR DIET: Gassy foods include cruciferous vegetables (broccoli, cauliflower, brussels sprouts, cabbage), onions, radishes, bananas, apricots, and whole

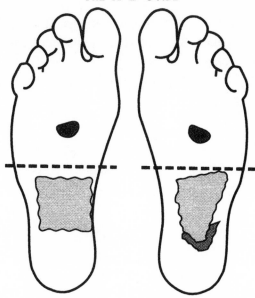

wheat flour. Many people (whether lactose-intolerant or not) have trouble digesting milk and milk products; try doing without them for a few days, and see if the problem clears up. Beans tend to be the worst offenders; however, the gas problem may be eliminated by soaking them overnight before cooking.

TRY CHARCOAL: Activated charcoal tablets (available at your pharmacy) can absorb a great deal of the gas. Always check with your physician about taking charcoal if you are taking medication for any reason, since charcoal can absorb the drug as well.

EAT SLOWLY: Sit down and enjoy your food. Chew every bite, and don't talk (and take in so much air) while you eat. Take rests between courses, and if you are satiated with the food you've eaten, skip the next course. (You can always eat dessert later.)

INCREASE FIBER SLOWLY: Fiber, a nutritive element that most Americans never eat enough of, gets the bowel to work hard and may prevent colon cancer and heart disease. However, it can be hard to digest. If you're adding fiber to your diet, do it in small increments, increasing the amount each week.

If neither reflexology nor any of the alternative therapies listed above alleviate your flatulence, consult your physician.

FRACTURES

The fall didn't seem awfully bad, but you landed right on your elbow, and the pain is excruciating. Or perhaps you turned a little oddly coming down the stairs. You thought you'd just twisted your ankle, but the X ray shows a nasty break.

A fracture may be clean (one break right through the bone or cartilage) or comminuted (the bone shatters in many pieces). Some fractures are stress fractures—that is, the fall or twist causes only a crack in the bone, which must be immobilized because it is painful even though it doesn't show up on an X ray. In an open or compound fracture the skin is broken, though there are closed fractures where the skin remains intact. A child, with bones that are more flexible than an adult's, may have a green stick fracture, where only one side of the bone is broken, or an impacted fracture, where the ends of bone are jammed together. In a complicated fracture, internal organs, blood vessels, and nerves may be damaged as well as the bone. The broken blood vessels around the area cause swelling at the site. Any compound fracture that has created an open wound is more serious, since it can become infected, and very often antibiotics are given as a prophylactic measure.

Most fractures are treated without surgery in a process called reduction: The doctor manipulates the bones so that they are positioned back together again and then immobilizes them with a hard or soft cast. A serious fracture involving damage to ligaments, tendons, or internal organs may require surgery, after which the bones are often held together with metal pins, plates, or rods. Depending on the problem, the appliances are either removed or left in the body.

AREAS TO TREAT/TYPES OF MANIPULATION

Work both feet completely first. Then work the area that corresponds to the injury on the opposite side of the body (see Chapter 3 for guidance).

PREVENTIVE MEASURES AND COMPLEMENTARY TREATMENTS

Reflexology works well in conjunction with other alternative therapies and commonsense measures. For example:

GET AN X RAY: If you've sustained a bad fall or twisted your ankle and it hurts so badly it's difficult or impossible to put weight on it, play it safe and have it X-rayed. Babying a fracture just doesn't work, and the bones won't grow back together if they aren't set properly. So don't be brave; get a professional opinion.

KEEP YOUR CAST DRY: Wear a plastic bag over your cast whenever you take a shower.

WEAR YOUR SLING: If you've injured your arm or hand, (particularly if it's on your primary side), it's tempting to try to use it as much as possible. But it's important to let the healing process take place, so keep your sling on.

EXERCISE THE AREA WHEN IT'S HEALED: While your fracture is kept in place with a cast or splint, the muscles around it don't get used. It's therefore very important to start slowly as soon as your doctor advises, exercising the atrophied muscles so that they can regain their former shape and strength.

Fractures must be treated in an emergency room or by your own physician. However, reflexology may provide additional relief while you are healing.

GALLSTONES

You may not think anything is wrong except lately it's harder to digest high-fat foods. You sometimes have some pain in the upper abdomen, and you've been nauseated without reason. Then one night after dinner it hits hard: a sharp pain in the upper right quadrant of your abdomen that goes all the way up to your shoulder. You may think you have the flu because of the fever and chills, but your yellowish complexion argues against that.

Gallstones are hard lumps of cholesterol mixed with calcium, blood, and bile (the fluid produced by the liver). They form either in the gallbladder itself or in the bile duct, which goes from the gallbladder to the intestine.

Individuals with high cholesterol are more prone to gallstones. As levels rise, and the bile combines with these fatty deposits, hard masses form. Some conditions that may adversely affect LDL levels are pregnancy, diabetes, obesity, liver disease, and some types of anemia. If you're a yo-yo dieter, always losing weight and then gaining it back, you're more at risk for gallstones; if you've had more than two babies, you're also at higher risk. Although experts don't know why, twice as many women as men over forty develop gallstones.

Half of those who develop gallstones have no symptoms. However, if the stones lodge in the bile duct, excruciating pain may result.

SYMPTOMS: Some people have no symptoms at all; others may experience flatulence and belching, acid indigestion, mild jaundice (a yellowing of the skin), and discomfort after meals. The symptom of a gallbladder attack, however, is acute and excruciating pain that may radiate from the upper abdomen to the back or right shoulder. The attack is caused by a gallstone lodging in the bile duct.

AREAS TO TREAT/TYPES OF MANIPULATION

Work both feet completely first. Then find the locations of the liver and gallbladder reflexes, and work them carefully (see Chapter 3 for guidance):

Liver/Gallbladder: Apply direct pressure to gallbladder; then glide up and to left across liver.

PREVENTIVE MEASURES AND COMPLEMENTARY TREATMENTS

Reflexology works well in conjunction with other alternative therapies and commonsense measures. For example:

REDUCE YOUR CHOLESTEROL: Although there are individuals who manufacture a great deal of cholesterol despite what they eat, it's always wise to reduce dietary intake. Select low-fat, no-fat, and low-cholesterol products.

GET SOME EXERCISE: Aerobic activity is a proven method of reducing LDL cholesterol. It will also trigger

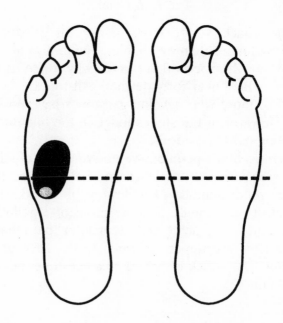

the release of beta-endorphins in your brain, those "feel-good" natural opiates that will help you stick to your diet.

Gallstones must be treated by a physician, and surgery may be necessary to remove the gallbladder. However, reflexology and alternative therapies can help reduce the inflammation and pain of this condition.

GLAUCOMA (SEE ALSO EYE PAIN, P. 132)

Your eye is hard and red; your vision is blurred. You kept thinking it was just age; you just don't see the way you should. There are halos around lights, and you have tunnel vision, unable to make out anything on the peripheries.

Glaucoma is a painful eye condition caused by increased pressure in the eyeball. This disease, which may be acute or chronic, occurs because the fluids within the eye can no longer drain as they should. In a normal eye the aqueous humor (eye fluid) flows between the anterior chamber of the eye in front of the lens and the posterior chamber behind the lens. The iris separates these two chambers.

But when glaucoma strikes, most commonly in individuals over forty, part of the iris blocks the way, so that the fluid stays in the anterior chamber. More fluid may be produced than can be absorbed by the veins in the eye, and this results in a buildup of pressure on the eyeball. It becomes hard and painful.

Chronic glaucoma develops gradually, as the passageway between the chambers is narrowed by the angle of drainage from one side to the other. Pressure in the eye rises gradually.

Acute glaucoma comes on quickly, when pressure in the anterior chamber suddenly presses the iris into the cornea, blocking the way so that fluid cannot drain into the posterior chamber.

Although there seems to be a predisposition in families for several members to develop the condition, the exact cause is not known. Steroid drug users are at higher risk (steroids change the levels of fluid throughout the body), as are those who have had histories of eye infections and cataracts.

symptoms: *Chronic:* You may see a vague white halo surrounding distant lights. Also, you may experience gradual deterioration of peripheral vision followed by foggy or blurred vision, difficulty adjusting from bright lights to dark, slight pain on one side of the eye.

Acute: You may have sudden excruciating eye pain, which may cause nausea and/or vomiting. Your vision will blur abruptly. MEDICAL ATTENTION IS NEEDED IMMEDIATELY IN ORDER TO PREVENT BLINDNESS.

AREAS TO TREAT/TYPES OF MANIPULATION

Work both feet completely first. Then find the locations of reflexes that correspond to these organs, and work in the following order (see Chapter 3 for guidance):

1. Eye/Ear: Apply direct circular pressure with thumb tip.
2. Neck: Using thumb and index finger, manipulate "necks" of toes thoroughly.
3. Kidneys: Apply direct pressure with thumb tip.

PREVENTIVE MEASURES AND COMPLEMENTARY TREATMENTS

Reflexology works well in conjunction with other alternative therapies and commonsense measures. For example:

GET REGULAR CHECKUPS: See an ophthalmologist or optometrist on a yearly basis for a glaucoma check.

Glaucoma must be treated by a physician, with medication, surgery, or both. However, reflexology and alternative therapies can help establish better accommodation to impaired vision.

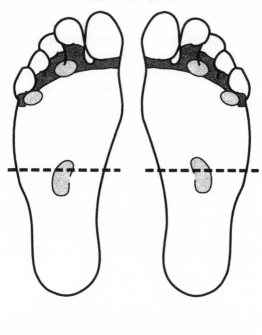

GOUT

Suddenly you're awakened by a searing pain in the joint of your big toe. You played a few sets of tennis earlier and then had more than a few drinks with some friends, but you can't figure this as part of a hangover. A few days later you're worse: The joint is inflamed, swollen, red, hot to the touch, and so excruciatingly painful you can't even put a sock on. You've been running a low-grade fever with chills, and your heart rate is going a mile a minute.

Gout is actually a form of arthritis, triggered by too much uric acid in the blood, so much that the kidneys can't process it as they normally do. The acid then crystallizes and collects in and around the joints, such as the big toe, ankle, knee, wrist, and elbow. These joints and their neighboring tendons consequently become inflamed and painful. Uric acid deposits may also collect in the kidneys, forming kidney stones (see Kidney Stones, p. 218).

SYMPTOMS: Sudden pain in a joint, often occurring in the middle of the night after excessive exercise or alcohol consumption. Later fever, swelling of joint, rapid heartbeat. Uric acid deposits can be detected under the skin in the hands, feet, elbows, and rims of the ears. Attacks usually occur within months of each other, but if the disease is not treated, the period between attacks shortens to weeks or days.

AREAS TO TREAT/TYPES OF MANIPULATION

Work both feet completely first. Then find the locations of reflexes that correspond to these organs, and work in the following order (see Chapter 3 for guidance):

1. Kidneys: Apply direct pressure with thumb tip.
2. Use reflex corresponding to affected area of body. Locate the area on general chart of foot, pages 30–31.

PREVENTIVE MEASURES AND COMPLEMENTARY TREATMENTS

Reflexology works well in conjunction with other alternative therapies and commonsense measures. For example:

CHANGE YOUR DIET: If you generally eat a lot of rich foods, this is the time to streamline your diet. Cut way down on protein—you might want to have meat, poultry, or fish in small portions every other day. Eliminate foods that increase the body's production of uric acid,

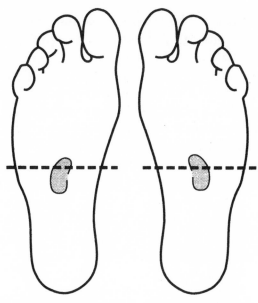

such as anchovies, herrings, mussels, sardines, sweet-breads, brains, liver, kidneys, and mincemeat.

You can also add cherries (fresh, canned, juice, or concentrate). Anecdotal evidence indicates that this fruit alleviates gout symptoms.

BAN THE BOOZE: Alcohol, particularly beer, raises uric acid levels and makes it more difficult for the body to excrete this acid in the urine.

TRY CHARCOAL: Activated charcoal taken by mouth (1/2 to 1 teaspoon four times daily) or as a poultice or bath (1/2 cup charcoal powder diluted with warm water) appears to soothe inflamed joints and draw toxins out of the body.

TAKE NSAIDS: Ibuprofen, a nonsteroidal anti-inflammatory drug, will bring down the swelling and pain. Take two four times daily, or consult your physician if this amount isn't enough to take the edge off. (CAUTION: Do not take aspirin, which can increase uric acid levels.)

TRY R.I.C.E.: Rest, ice, compression, and elevation

make a good combination for painful joints. You can use this formula as you practice your reflexology and other alternative treatments.

If neither reflexology nor any of the alternative therapies listed above alleviate the pain associated with gout, consult your physician, who will prescribe medication to relieve inflammation or uricosuric drugs to balance uric acid levels in the blood.

Hay Fever (see also Allergies, p. 48)

It's that time of year again. It doesn't matter whether you're indoors or out, you just sneeze your head off. Your eyes and nose are red and watery; you feel miserable.

Hay fever, a type of rhinitis (an inflammation of the mucous membranes in the nose), occurs in certain sensitive individuals in the spring, summer, and fall, when trees, grass, flowers, and weeds give off their pollens. Some people develop a nonallergic type of hay fever that lasts all year long. With this type of rhinitis, the body produces antigens to dust, mold, spores, feathers, or animal dander.

This condition may begin in childhood and continue, or it may start up in later life, sometimes when you change environments and are living in an area with different foliage from that which you've been used to.

SYMPTOMS: Sneezing, headache, runny nose, itchy and watery eyes, itching inside the nose and at the roof of the mouth, insomnia, fatigue.

AREAS TO TREAT/TYPES OF MANIPULATION

Work both feet completely first. Then find the locations of reflexes that correspond to these organs, and work in the following order (see Chapter 3 for guidance):

1. Adrenals: Apply direct pressure with thumb tip.
2. Reproductive System: Apply gradual circular pressure with thumb tip and pad to reflexes for ovaries and uterus (females) or prostate and testes (male).
3. Pituitary: Apply direct pressure with thumb tip.
4. Head/Sinus: Using the tip of the thumb, first work the tips of all the toes, using a circular motion; then work all around the whole toe.
5. Neck: Using thumb and index finger, manipulate "necks" of the toes thoroughly.
6. Ileocecal Valve: Apply direct pressure with thumb tip.

PREVENTIVE MEASURES AND COMPLEMENTARY TREATMENTS

Reflexology works well in conjunction with other alternative therapies and commonsense measures. For example:

STAY IN COOL, DRY AIR: Air-conditioning is almost mandatory, particularly in your bedroom and car. You should also invest in a dehumidifier and an industrial-quality air cleaner that plugs into your central heating and cooling system.

WEAR A MASK WHEN YOU GARDEN: If you just love the outdoors, you'll probably risk the symptoms. But you can reduce them a little by wearing a paper mask (found in hardware stores) as you work.

GIVE YOURSELF A CATPROOF, FLOWERPROOF ROOM: Your family may adore the family pet, and they may delight in a beautiful bouquet on the dining room table. Your life

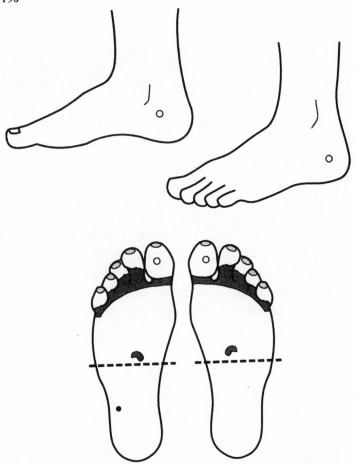

will be easier, however, if you make one room your sanctuary. Keep it air-conditioned, uncarpeted, and scrupulously clean, and close the door every time you leave it.

TRY VISUALIZING: The mind can work wonders to keep the immune system from producing antibodies to various allergens. (This has been proved in individuals with multiple personality disorder; one of the personalities may be highly allergic while the others are not.) So give yourself twenty minutes a day to imagine that you are walking through a beautiful grassy field strewn with wildflowers. You are encased in an invisible protective bubble that no one can see but that screens out any foreign element that might cause you problems. Breathe deeply now, inhaling the perfume of the flowers. Enjoy the experience of sitting in the lush grass. Tell yourself that each day you will be able to tolerate a longer period of exposure, and you will truly begin to enjoy the outdoors as you never have before.

Since hay fever is seasonal, you should be using reflexology and alternative treatments preventively, just before the pollens emerge. You should consult your doctor if you are having shortness of breath or wheezing. He or she may recommend antihistamines (to dry up your nasal passages) or a short course of corticosteroid drugs to reduce inflammation.

Headaches/Migraines

It may feel like a steel band right around your head, a throbbing pulse at your temple, or a sick feeling in the stomach that connects up with every nerve in your brain. You want to lie down in a dark room and escape the world; any sound, any touch is like chalk on a blackboard to you.

Although the brain itself doesn't feel pain, the nerves within the arteries and veins that supply blood to the brain are very sensitive. The nerve endings also produce pain-giving substances called prostaglandins that travel from the eyes, ears, nose, and skin to the brain. Tension and fatigue can shift the pressure, as can external causes like eyestrain, noise, lack of sleep, or a hangover.

The two basic forms of headache are tension headaches and vascular headaches (which include both migraines and cluster headaches).

Tension headaches are caused by a contraction of the skeletal muscles around the face, forehead, and the back of the neck. When the muscles contract, their supply of oxygen is reduced, and toxins build up in them and cause pain.

Because the blood vessels contract with this type of headache, warmth is often applied to open them up.

Migraine headaches are most prevalent in women and result from a dilation of blood vessels in the scalp and head. The pain is usually pulsing or throbbing, is one-sided, and can last from four to seventy-two hours. Because the blood vessels expand with this type of headache, cold is often applied to reduce them.

A migraine is a type of nervous system overexcitability. As there is a change in the regulation of blood flow throughout the head and body, the neurons become out of balance. Various triggers can cause a migraine; certain types of food like aged cheese and red wine, noise, or radical shifts in barometric pressure will do it. An unfortunate side effect is that a migraine effectively shuts down your brain's ability to produce endorphins, the natural opiates that stop pain.

Cluster headaches always occur in men and come in cycles. They often strike daily or every other day for one to three months (some men may have as many as four to eight a day), and then they mercifully stop for a few months before resuming again. Like migraines, the pain of these headaches is due to the expansion of blood vessels, but there is a hormonal component to them as well.

SYMPTOMS: All headaches are miserable, but they are miserable in different ways.

Tension Headaches: usually produce a dull pain that encompasses the whole head (or at least both sides) and is often described as a band of steel around the forehead. Headaches caused by eyestrain, fever, or sinus infection may have the same symptoms.

Migraine Headaches: give throbbing or pulsing pain on one side only. The "classic" migraine is often preceded by an aura, or a feeling that something is about to happen. The "common" migraine does not give the sufferer this leeway, unfortunately. The headache often brings with it extreme nausea and light sensitivity. Sometimes the migraine sufferer will see flashing lights, zigzagging light patterns, or have blank spaces in his or her visual field.

Throbbing pain is also present in headaches caused by hangovers and those caused by hypertension.

Cluster Headaches: reputed to be the most exquisite pain that exists. There have been suicides attributed to this type of headache. Medication is almost always necessary. However, reflexology can assist in alleviating tension throughout the body and removing energy blockages that may start to break up the headache cycle.

AREAS TO TREAT/TYPES OF MANIPULATION

Work both feet completely first. Then find the locations of reflexes that correspond to these organs, and work in the following order (see Chapter 3 for guidance):

1. Head/Sinus: Using the tip of the thumb, first work the tips of all the toes, using a circular motion; then work all around the whole toe.
2. Neck: Using thumb and index finger, manipulate "necks" of toes thoroughly.

3. Solar Plexus: With thumb tip, apply gradual pressure in the middle of the reflex, and work out to the edges.

4. Tailbone (Coccyx): Holding the foot with one hand, glide the thumb tip of your other hand from the top of the heel to the bottom of the heel.

PREVENTIVE MEASURES AND COMPLEMENTARY TREATMENTS

Reflexology works well in conjunction with other alternative therapies and commonsense measures. For example:

PRACTICE RELAXATION TECHNIQUES: By learning meditation, visualization, and directed breathing, you can stop a headache in its tracks or "move" it out of your head. Take twenty minutes a day to sit, with no goals in mind, whether or not you have a headache, and pay attention to your inhalation and exhalation. Don't attempt to force other thoughts from your mind, but rather, let them pass through, as though they were passengers walking through the train car in which you're seated.

If you do have a headache, imagine it as an object that you are going to wrap up in a package and discard. Visualize the paper and string, carefully cover the entire headache, tie it up, and secure the string. Now picture a hole in the top of your head through which you will guide the string and, after it, the package. When everything is out, close up the hole in your head. Now you can imagine throwing the headache in the garbage, burying it in the ground, or shredding it into tiny pieces.

AVOID ALCOHOL AND TOBACCO: Alcohol increases blood flow to the head and dilates blood vessels; nicotine does the same. Don't consume these substances if you want to stay headache-free.

TRY A PASSIONATE EMBRACE: Sexual stimulation increases the flow in the brain of neurotransmitters that

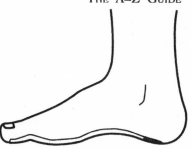

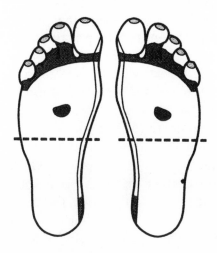

block pain. Also, when you're aroused, you have more blood flow in the genital area, and that makes less blood available to move upward and pound in your forehead and scalp. So instead of responding, "Not tonight, darling, I have a headache," when your partner is interested, switch to "Yes, darling, tonight's the night!"

BREATHE SOME SEA AIR: Negatively charged ions have a healing effect on mind and body. In nature the ratio of positive to negative ions is five to one, but in polluted environments and big cities there just aren't enough negative ions. A study at Columbia University found that headache sufferers who took a half-hour walk by the beach tended to feel better than those who stayed indoors. The sea air really does make a difference.

STAY OUT OF THE SUN: The beating rays of the sun dry up the fluids that help regulate pressure and balance in the brain. As drier blood vessels rub against one another, they create unpleasant friction that can trigger a headache. So stay in the shade, and wear a hat and sunglasses to keep away from the sun's effects.

GET SOME THERAPY: Myofacial release and craniosacral therapy are two forms of body work related to both chiropractic and massage that have great benefits for headache sufferers. The practitioners of these therapies use gentle touch to find areas of blockage and then release the blocks with directed pressure to those areas.

WATCH WHAT YOU EAT: Certain foods contain chemicals that can spark a migraine. Be sure to avoid monosodium glutamate (MSG) and foods containing tyramine, an organic compound found in aged cheese, deli meats, soy sauce, eggplant, figs, and products made with yeast.

If you have a headache that refuses to respond to reflexology, the alternative therapies listed above, or over-the-counter medications, or if you've had persistent headaches over a period of weeks, see your physician.

HEARING LOSS

If "What did you say?" is becoming your most frequent phrase, you may be experiencing hearing loss.

There are several different reasons for the problem. There may be a defect in the outer or middle ear preventing sound transmission from reaching the hearing center in the brain (conductive deafness). This condition may be congenital (you are born with this defect) or may result from an accident or injury to the eardrum or bones in the ear. A second type of problem occurs when the inner ear or the auditory nerve or the brain center that processes hearing is damaged (sensorineural deafness). Certain illnesses (mumps, meningitis, multiple sclerosis, or Ménière's disease) may cause this type of hearing loss, as can a hemorrhage or blood clot in the inner ear, the side effects of drugs, or prolonged exposure to high-decibel sound. A third condition, mixed deafness, is a combination of the other two types. Yet another condition that damages hearing but that is reparable by surgery is otosclerosis. Here an abnormal bone growth over the middle ear prevents clear sound from passing through.

One of my clients, Will, had a blockage in his left ear, which may have been only a long-term buildup of wax but may also have been a result of mixed deafness. It had given him partial hearing loss and was beginning to affect his balance (which is affected by shifting fluids in the ear). He was also in a lot of discomfort much of the time. In my treatments I concentrated on both ears, eyes, sinuses, and neck. We'd had about five sessions together when Will told me he didn't know whether his hearing was any better, but he sure felt more relaxed from the reflexology. With this, he yawned, his left ear popped, and the blockage cleared. He never had a recurrence of the problem.

SYMPTOMS: At first there is an inability to pick up certain words, and as hearing loss progresses, it becomes increasingly difficult to hear any sound (particularly high-pitched sounds) well. With certain conditions, there may also be a ringing in the ears. The ability to hear eventually deteriorates so that only loud lower-pitched sounds come through.

AREAS TO TREAT/TYPES OF MANIPULATION

Work both feet completely first. Then find the locations of reflexes that correspond to these organs and work in the following order (see Chapter 3 for guidance):

1. Eye/Ear: Apply direct circular pressure with thumb tip.
2. Neck: Using thumb and index finger, manipulate "necks" of toes thoroughly.

PREVENTIVE MEASURES AND COMPLEMENTARY TREATMENTS

Reflexology works well in conjunction with other alternative therapies and commonsense measures. For example:

CLEAN YOUR EARS: Wax is a normal secretion in the ear. However, when it becomes too abundant, it may harden and present hearing problems. A good preventive measure is a weekly gentle cleaning with hydrogen peroxide on a Q-Tip. Be very careful not to stick the Q-Tip too far inside the ear. (Wax that has collected beyond this point will have to be removed by a physician.)

REALLY LISTEN: Sometimes people with hearing problems develop listening problems as well. Because the sound doesn't come through clearly, they often stop trying to make sense of words. A good exercise is to focus on the speaker and the topic and clear your mind of anything that would prevent a complete transmission of the message.

GET TESTED: If you are having problems, you should consult an audiologist, who will give you appropriate

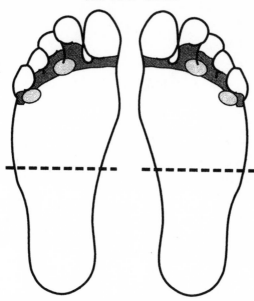

tests to determine the degree of hearing loss and whether it's in one ear or both.

USE A HEARING AID IF YOU NEED ONE: The new devices on the market are really tiny, and although no hearing aid is perfect (it amplifies all sound instead of just the sound you want to hear), it's better than not understanding what's going on around you. The audiologist (see p. 164) will be able to recommend a specialist in audiometry to find the type that's right for you.

If reflexology and the alternative therapies listed have not resolved your hearing problems, you should consult your family physician, who may refer you to a hearing specialist.

✳

HEARTBURN

"My chest is on fire" is the only thought you have when you've got heartburn, or pyrosis. That uncomfortable burning feeling right behind the breastbone, rising up to the throat, is often accompanied by belching, nausea, and a full feeling in the upper abdomen. The pain may be so intense you could swear it's angina. (Many people who have angina unfortunately ignore their real problem for years, stating that they just get heartburn a lot.)

Some people claim they could spit fire; others just want to lie down until it goes away. Caused by eating too quickly, exercising after eating, wearing constricting clothing while eating, or normal eating combined with a faulty digestive tract, heartburn is a common complaint of anyone suffering from acid reflux—a slight backup of stomach acid into the esophagus. One of the chemicals found in digestive enzymes is hydrochloric acid, an exceptionally harsh substance that can eat right through leather.

The stomach has a protective lining that keeps it safe from this acid; the esophagus does not, however, and this is why the pain can be so severe. The more the stomach fills up, the more acid is likely to be displaced and rise into the esophagus.

AREAS TO TREAT/TYPES OF MANIPULATION

Work both feet completely first. Then find the locations of reflexes that correspond to these organs (see Chapter 3 for guidance):

1. Throat: Apply gradual direct pressure on the reflex point (CAUTION: This can be painful.)
2. Stomach: Apply gradual circular pressure with thumb tip and pad.
3. Solar Plexus: With thumb tip, apply gradual pressure in the middle of reflex, and work out to the edges.
4. Colon: Beginning on the right foot, glide the thumb tip from the ileocecal valve up the ascending colon, across the transverse colon, to the inside edge of the foot.

    Continue with the left foot. Glide the thumb left to right across the transverse colon, down the descending colon, and end with a slight hook upward at sigmoid colon.

PREVENTIVE MEASURES AND COMPLEMENTARY TREATMENTS

Reflexology works well in conjunction with other alternative therapies and commonsense measures. For example:

EAT IN MODERATION: It's vital that you watch not only what you eat but how you eat it. If you can possibly treat eating as a sensory experience, you will find that you stop consuming your food while standing up or in front of the television set or in your car. The more you eat mindfully—that is, thinking about the benefits of the nourishment you're taking in—the better your body's ability to process those nutrients.

TAKE AN ANTACID: As long as you don't make it a daily habit, you can take an over-the-counter preparation to alleviate the pain. But if your chronic heartburn persists for more than two weeks, you should stop self-medicating and get a thorough checkup, just to make sure that your heartburn isn't a symptom of a more serious condition.

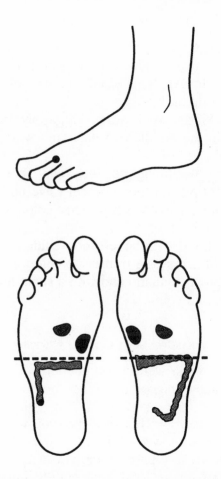

PROP UP YOUR HEAD: The more upright you can stay, the better, since gravity will work for you and keep the acid from rising up. If you're really in pain and want to lie down, keep your head and chest slightly elevated.

ELIMINATE CAFFEINE AND NICOTINE: Coffee, tea, sodas, and chocolate all contain caffeine, which is a stimulant and contains other chemicals that irritate the esophagus. Smoking—in addition to being a life-threatening risk—also irritates the mucous membranes of the throat and esophagus.

WEAR LOOSE CLOTHING: It doesn't help to squeeze into tight jeans or wear your belt pulled to its extreme. If you're prone to heartburn, and particularly at mealtime, slip into something more comfortable.

TRY AN HERBAL REMEDY: The best herbs for heartburn are ginger bitters (available as a liquid extract in some supermarkets and specialty food stores and containing gentian root, goldenseal, wormwood, and fennel. Take two capsules or half a dropper of extract after meals).

If reflexology and other alternative therapies have not alleviated your heartburn after two weeks, if you have pain on swallowing or pain referred to your shoulder, or if you vomit blood or have black stools, consult your physician. It's possible that the pain is due to an ulcer, which must be treated medically.

Heart Disease

That feeling of squeezing, strangulating pain right in the center of your chest is terrifying, but mystifying, because it goes away if you sit down and rest. Or perhaps you suddenly feel your heart skip a beat or add several beats.

There are many disorders of the heart and circulatory system, some of which you may be born with and others of which may develop as you age. Heart disease is the number one killer of men and women in America, and it is vital that we all understand how to care for the heart, that hollow muscular organ that pumps 1.8 million barrels of blood through our bodies over the course of an average lifetime.

The most common type of heart disease is coronary artery disease, or atherosclerosis, a condition caused by the development of fatty deposits, known as plaque, on the inside of the coronary arteries that encircle the heart. As it becomes more difficult for blood to pass from the heart to the lungs through the narrowed passageways, the tissues don't receive enough oxygen, and pain mid-chest (angina) is often present. When the arteries become so blocked that blood cannot pass through, a heart attack may result. You are more likely to suffer from this condition if you have high blood pressure and high levels of LDL cholesterol, if you smoke, and if you have a family history of heart disease.

Hypertension (high blood pressure) is another common form of heart disease. In this condition the heart has to pump harder to get blood through the arteries, working against increased resistance as it tries to pass through the narrowed arteries. The higher-pressure blood flow—similar to a high-pressure water hose—creates shear stresses on artery walls, which may break apart already existing plaques. This can start up the body's clotting system and lead to heart attacks or strokes.

A stroke is a cardiac event that takes place when sufficient blood doesn't reach the brain. As a result, brain cells die or are damaged so that they can't perform their normal functions involved with moving, seeing, hearing, or thinking.

Cardiac arrhythmias occur because of a disruption in the electrical activity of the heart. You may have too many beats, not enough beats, or the walls of either the top or bottom chambers of the heart may begin to contract at irregular intervals.

In mitral valve prolapse, a seemingly hereditary disorder almost exclusively seen in women, one of the valves of the heart (which open and close to allow blood to flow in only one direction) is enlarged and "floppy." The valve doesn't shut properly; that means blood flows backward, causing a classic clicking sound.

Congestive heart failure occurs when the heart cannot meet the oxygen and metabolic needs of the body. The heart weakens and can't pump blood to feed the various organs and tissues. This creates a problem of salt and water retention and lung congestion.

SYMPTOMS: The various problems each have their own symptoms:

Atherosclerosis: The most common symptom is angina, pain in the center of the chest that sometimes radiates down the left side of the body. Angina usually starts up when you're active and goes away when you sit down and rest (although there are types of angina that are not alleviated by rest). You may also experience shortness of breath or great fatigue. A less typical symptom is a feeling of fullness, like indigestion, or an achiness across the upper back. The most dangerous symptom of atherosclerosis, of course, is a heart attack.

Hypertension: Very often there are no symptoms. In some cases you may experience headaches or shortness of breath.

Stroke: Symptoms include weakness and numbness in limbs, on the face, or down one side of the body. You may suddenly lose vision in one eye or be unable to speak or understand speech. Other symptoms are dizziness, falling, and loss of consciousness.

Cardiac Arrhythmias: You may have irregular heartbeats—skipping a beat or having more beats than normal. Other common symptoms are palpitations, the feeling of the heart pounding and bumping in the chest. They may go on for hours, indicating that the rhythm of the heart is disturbed.

Mitral Valve Prolapse: You may feel chest pain (different from angina), which is characterized by a brief stabbing pain to the left of the breastbone that occurs at intervals. You may also experience palpitations, dizziness, numbness, fatigue, and panic attacks.

Congestive Heart Failure: Symptoms are shortness of breath (which may actually rouse you from sleep with a feeling that you can't breathe), coughing or wheezing, swelling of body parts caused by water retention, rapid heartbeat, and enormous fatigue.

Areas to Treat/Types of Manipulation

Work both feet completely first. Then find the locations of reflexes that correspond to these organs (see Chapter 3 for guidance):

1. Heart: Work with thumb tip, using circular motion.
2. Lungs: With tip and edge of thumb, work up and down and left to right.
3. Adrenals: Apply direct pressure with thumb tip.
4. Sigmoid Colon: Apply direct pressure with thumb tip.
5. Solar Plexus: With thumb tip, apply gradual pressure in the middle of reflex, and work out to the edges.

Preventive Measures and Complementary Treatments

Reflexology works well in conjunction with other alternative therapies and commonsense measures. For example:

CUT THE FAT: Clinical proof of reversing heart disease has been shown with a diet containing only 10 percent of its calories in fat. Since most Americans eat about 37 to 40 percent of their diet in fat, this is a drastic nutritional decision. If you can stay away from eating anything that walks, swims, crawls, or flies (basically a

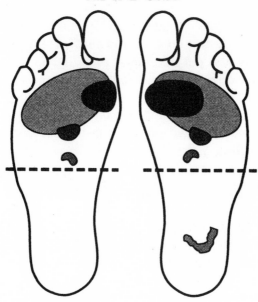

vegetarian diet without dairy products), you'll be on the road to lower cholesterol, triglycerides (another type of fat), and blood pressure.

GET OUT AND MOVE: Studies have shown that exercise raises HDL cholesterol (the "good" cholesterol that helps keep plaque off arteries) and lowers LDL cholesterol. It also triggers the production of beta-endorphins in the brain, those natural opiates that make you feel so good you want to stick with your low-fat diet.

STOP SMOKING: Nicotine stimulates the release of epinephrine, which raises blood pressure and constricts blood vessels. Toxins in cigarettes leave lesions on coronary artery walls, which make it easier for plaque to be deposited there. Cigarettes can also trigger spasms in the coronary arteries, which can cause permanent damage to the heart. The best thing you can do for your heart is never to pick up this insidious habit; the next best thing is to stop now.

REDUCE YOUR STRESS: Stress itself causes blood vessels

to constrict and triggers the release of hormones (adrenaline, noradrenaline, and cortisol) that raise LDL cholesterol and put additional pressure on the arteries. A structured program of some stress management therapy, such as meditation, visualization, yoga, tai chi chuan, biofeedback, or a support group, won't necessarily make you calm, but it will teach you to keep stress under control.

All forms of heart disease must be managed by a physician. Medication or surgery may be necessary in advanced stages of these conditions. However, reflexology and alternative therapies can keep the body in balance so that conventional medical treatment will work more quickly and effectively.

HEMORRHOIDS

You can't sit down, and sometimes you can't stand up either. It's not clear whether the pain or the itching is worse. Going to the bathroom is agony, and the whole thing is too embarrassing to discuss. This had to be where we got the expression "What a pain in the ***!"

Hemorrhoids, or piles, are swollen veins inside or just outside the wall of the anus. When these veins become inflamed, they swell, causing itching and pain. Hemorrhoids develop because of repeated pressure on the area when you bear down to pass hardened stools. This unpleasant situation may occur because you have a sedentary lifestyle (and enough blood isn't flowing in the area) or because you postpone having a bowel movement and consequently the stools lose moisture and are more difficult to pass. Hemorrhoids can also develop during pregnancy and in people who are obese or have liver disease. They may also occur to those who abuse laxatives.

What you eat of course determines what you eliminate. If your diet is made up of refined foods and you don't have enough fiber, you may be chronically constipated, and this can lead to the development of hemorrhoids.

These swollen varicose veins, which may be internal or external, may bleed during or after a bowel movement and may begin to itch or hurt at any time. The internal hemorrhoids may prolapse, falling down out of the anus and appearing as small brown skin "tags" that can be manually inserted back inside. External hemorrhoids, formed from the rupture of an interior rectal vein, show up as blood blisters, or hematomas, around the anus.

SYMPTOMS: Itching and pain during and after bowel movements; bleeding after a bowel movement; the development of external "tags" or hematomas around the anus.

AREAS TO TREAT/TYPES OF MANIPULATION

Work both feet completely first. Then find the locations of reflexes that correspond to these organs, and work in the following order (see Chapter 3 for guidance):

1. Hip: Work thumb edge all around lower edge of outer anklebone.
2. Lower Back (Lumbar Spine): Glide thumb tip down the inside of the foot from the base of the ball to the top of the heel.
3. Sigmoid Colon: Apply direct pressure to reflex with thumb tip.

4. Solar Plexus: With thumb tip, apply gradual pressure in the middle of reflex, and work out to the edges.

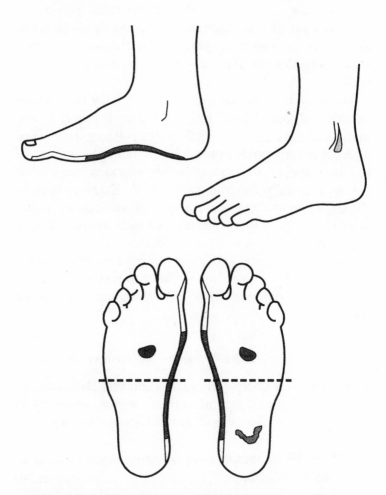

PREVENTIVE MEASURES AND COMPLEMENTARY TREATMENTS

Reflexology works well in conjunction with other alternative therapies and commonsense measures. For example:

ADD ROUGHAGE: Eat only whole foods, including bran, prunes, and cereals with psyllium seeds. Increase your consumption of fresh fruits (with skins on) and vegetables, and cut down on processed, high-fat, and high-protein foods.

You may find that highly spiced foods are irritating to your intestines. Try bland foods for a while, and see if they help.

CUT OUT COFFEE, BEER, AND COLAS: The caffeine in the first and the bubbles in the second and third also irritate your system. Switch to pure springwater, fruit juices, and herbal teas, and see if you're not more comfortable.

SIT IN A BATH: A sitz bath filled with warm water will soothe your hemorrhoids and alleviate itching.

CUT OUT LAXATIVES; USE A STOOL SOFTENER: Stool softeners will change the quality of the feces and make elimination easier and more pleasant. Avoid laxatives, which will keep your system from getting on its own natural course. If you're eating right, you won't need a laxative anyway.

USE WIPES: Tucks medicated pads are more gentle to your bottom than any toilet paper; they contain witch hazel and aloe, both soothing herbs. You may also put a little witch hazel on a cotton ball, and apply it directly to your anus between bowel movements.

Reflexology and alternative treatments will be able to keep most hemorrhoids under control. However, if you are bleeding excessively after bowel movements, or if you are in a great deal of pain, you should see your physician for an examination. Bleeding can cause anemia, and it may also be a symptom of colon cancer, so it's best to get your hemorrhoids checked out.

HERNIA

You cough, and suddenly a part of your stomach bulges out. For a while you quickly push it back in, but it becomes harder to bend over, to walk, even to stand still.

A hernia is a rupture of the abdominal wall that allows organs or parts of organs to protrude. There are several different types. Inguinal hernia, which is more common in men than in women, is a rupture in the groin. With an indirect inguinal hernia, a part of the peritoneum (the lining of the abdominal cavity) protrudes through the inguinal canal. When you cough or strain to defecate, the abdominal contents swell and protrude out. With a direct inguinal hernia, the abdominal organs push through the weakened muscles of the wall of the groin. This condition is greatly complicated if a loop of intestine slips down toward the groin and becomes twisted (strangulated hernia), cutting off the blood supply to that part of the gut.

Scrotal hernia, also a male problem, occurs when an inguinal hernia protrudes all the way down to the scrotum.

A femoral hernia, which is more common in women, is a rupture in the femoral canal at the top of the leg. The abdominal contents may bulge out over the thigh.

For a hiatal hernia, see below.

SYMPTOMS: A lump or bulging in the groin or upper leg area that may occur during coughing or straining at stools. The abdominal content can be felt and initially is "reducible"—that is, it can usually be pushed back inside. If the hernia is substantial or becomes strangulated, cutting off blood supply, it may cause nausea and pain on bending over, walking, or standing.

AREAS TO TREAT/TYPES OF MANIPULATION

Work both feet completely first. Then find the locations of reflexes that correspond to these organs, and work in the following order (see Chapter 3 for guidance):

1. Stomach: Apply gradual circular pressure with thumb tip and pad.
2. Solar Plexus: With thumb tip, apply gradual pressure in the middle of reflex, and work out to the edges.

PREVENTIVE MEASURES AND COMPLEMENTARY TREATMENTS

Reflexology works well in conjunction with other alternative therapies and commonsense measures. For example:

DON'T LIFT HEAVY OBJECTS: Picking up heavy weights, shoveling snow, attempting to lift windows that are stuck shut all can contribute to the development of a hernia. Let someone else do the work!

WEAR A SUPPORT BELT, AND BEND YOUR KNEES: If you absolutely have to do any lifting, wear a support belt (available in hardware stores and home repair centers). Always bend your knees and keep your head in line with your torso and hips when you lift.

Reflexology and commonsense measures can help support the stomach and groin area. Even after hernias have developed, they can often be pushed back inside manually and in other cases can be managed by the use of a truss. However, if you are having extreme pain in your gut, you should consult a doctor immediately. An

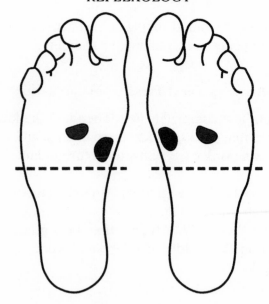

untreated strangulated hernia can lead to a serious infection of the stomach cavity.

HIATAL HERNIA

You feel a fullness in your chest after eating. You really wouldn't think anything of it except that the feeling gets worse when you bend over or lie down.

A hiatal or diaphragmatic hernia is a protrusion of the stomach above the diaphragm into the chest. Normally, when you swallow, your food passes from the throat to the esophagus and from there through a tight muscular band called a hiatus into the stomach. If this band loses its elasticity, pressure from below—a pregnancy, a tight belt, obesity, bending over, coughing, or straining—allows the top part of the stomach to slide through this relaxed opening.

A more serious variation of this hernia is the rolling hiatal hernia (paraesophageal hernia). In this condition a portion of the stomach and stomach lining roll up through the hiatus. The herniated section can get stuck in the chest, and blood supply can be shut off to a portion of the stomach, causing internal bleeding.

SYMPTOMS: Usually none other than a sense of fullness in the chest after eating.

AREAS TO TREAT/TYPES OF MANIPULATION

Work both feet completely first. Then find the locations of reflexes that correspond to these organs, and work in the following order (see Chapter 3 for guidance):

1. Solar Plexus: With thumb tip, apply gradual pressure in the middle of reflex, and work out to the edges.
2. Adrenals: Apply direct pressure with thumb tip.

PREVENTIVE MEASURES AND COMPLEMENTARY TREATMENTS

Reflexology works well in conjunction with other alternative therapies and commonsense measures. For example:

EAT SLOWLY AND REASONABLY: It's important to allow your body enough time to chew, swallow, and digest your food. This means sitting down to a meal, rather than eating standing up, walking, or in the car, and making each meal a leisurely and pleasant experience.

LOSE WEIGHT IF YOU HAVE TO: If you are more than 20 percent over your weight range as determined by life insurance tables, you are putting a strain on your gastro-

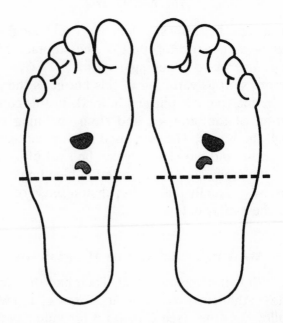

intestinal system as well as your heart. A sensible diet and exercise plan, monitored by your physician, will help you lose weight and remove pressure that may be exacerbating your hiatal hernia.

DON'T WEAR TIGHT CLOTHES: Tight jeans and belts constrict the diaphragm, making it even harder to digest properly. Even if you don't have a hiatal hernia, it's vital to give your internal organs the room to do their job properly. Go up a jean size, and loosen that belt!

Reflexology and commonsense measures may allow the various organ systems to accommodate to a weakened hiatus. Surgery is deemed necessary only in the most severe cases or with paraesophageal hernias.

HIP DISORDERS

You balance your groceries on them; you switch from one to the other when you've been standing too long; you rely on them to hold you up. The hips, more than the legs, seem like the foundation of the body because they stabilize you and hold all your weight. So when one gives out on you, it feels like a betrayal. The hip joint, strategically placed between the torso and lower body, can become a painful crutch to lean on.

The hip, the largest joint in the body, is designed to take the weight of the whole body so that you can stand, walk, and run efficiently and comfortably. The architecture of the hip is a ball and socket: The thighbone fits into a cup-shaped cavity (the acetabulum) in the pelvic girdle. The design of the socket is to face outward, away from the body, so that we can balance both legs as we walk.

To complete the assembly, there is cartilage over the head of the femur, lining the acetabulum, and synovial fluid to lubricate the joint so that it can swivel and bend easily. This fluid is secreted by the synovial membranes that make a tight seal around the joint itself. There are also several layers of fatty tissue that pad the joint to take the shock of impact as we move. Several different muscles, one running from the spine to the femur and the other from the pelvis to the femur, as well as other "helper" muscles in the thigh allow maximum flexibility of this joint.

SYMPTOMS: Various hip disorders will create different types of pain and disability:

Congenital Dislocation: Some babies are born with

their hips out of alignment or with a congenital instability. (The hip will be unstable if the head of the femur moves too easily out of the acetabulum.) This problem is generally treated by using metal braces on the hips and legs to keep them spread apart. (Less serious problems are sometimes treated by using two diapers at a time instead of one, again to train the legs to fall apart.)

Arthritis (see also Arthritis, p. 62): This term is a catchphrase for more than a hundred rheumatic diseases. Warning signs of both rheumatoid arthritis and osteoarthritis (the most common adult varieties) are pain, swelling, stiffness, or problems moving one or more joints. In rheumatoid arthritis the synovial membranes become inflamed, and the inflammation over time can cause chronic pain and deformity of the joint. With osteoarthritis the cartilage around the bone breaks down, and inflammation is caused by the rubbing of bone on bone.

Degenerative Joint Disease: In this condition the bony tissue at the top of the femur starts to disintegrate. The symptoms are sharp pains in the hip and possibly the knee and difficulty walking.

Osteoporosis: This condition of bone demineralization is common in postmenopausal women and in elderly men and women. Because the neck of the hip is so narrow, it is a likely place for a break, and it's common for individuals to fracture the bone and then to put their weight on it, causing a fall. (The fall didn't cause the break; the hip was broken before.)

Problems with Hip Replacement: Problems can arise even with a stainless steel and titanium hip that has replaced a badly broken human hip. During surgery, blood vessels may be damaged, cutting down on the ability of the wound to heal properly. The worse the break was and the older the patient is, the more likely it is that the artificial hip won't "take" well.

AREAS TO TREAT/TYPES OF MANIPULATION

Work both feet completely first. Then find the locations of reflexes that correspond to these organs, and work in the following order (see Chapter 3 for guidance):

1. Lymph Glands: Work thumb tip and pad gently back and forth across the area.
2. Groin: Apply firm thumb pressure throughout the bottom of the heel.
3. Hip/Sciatic Nerve: Work the edge of the thumb all around the lower edge of the anklebone.
4. Lower Back (Lumbar Spine): Glide thumb tip down the inside of the foot from the base of the ball to the top of the heel.
5. Knee: Work the end of the thumb all around the reflex point—the fifth metatarsal bone on the outside of each foot.

PREVENTIVE MEASURES AND COMPLEMENTARY TREATMENTS

Reflexology works well in conjunction with other alternative therapies and commonsense measures. For example:

PRACTICE YOGA OR TAI CHI CHUAN: The gentlest postures of either of these two types of meditative exercise can give you greater awareness of your range of movement. By working with an experienced teacher, you will learn to align your ankle, knee, hip, waist, shoulder, and head as you hold a dynamic posture or move through space. Other forms of body work, such as Feldenkrais or Alexander technique, can also teach you where you hold tension in your hips.

GET A MASSAGE: Both Swedish massage and shiatsu massage offer pain relief and greater relaxation. Sports massage is a growing field, and there are many excellent

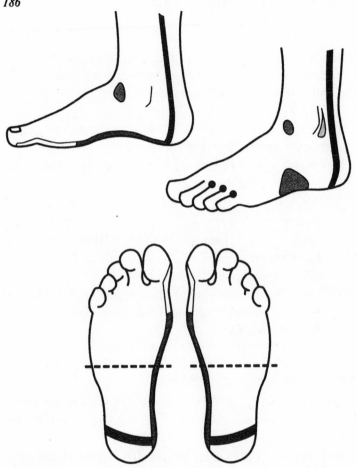

practitioners who know exactly what to do to alleviate pain in your joints and muscles.

WALK AROUND: Put on a good pair of walking shoes, and get out daily, starting with a walk to the corner and building up to half a mile over several weeks. Make sure you balance your weight evenly between both legs; try not to favor the affected side.

If neither reflexology nor any of the alternative measures provide relief, and if you have constant pain in your hip, consult a physician.

Hypertension (High Blood Pressure)

You may not think that anything is the matter except for the enormous tension in your body. When you get angry, your face is red, and it's hard to breathe. You get killer headaches, even when you're not particularly stressed.

High blood pressure is caused by a resistance to blood flow that occurs when the diameter of the small blood vessels narrows. If you have high blood pressure, your heart has to work harder and use more oxygen to move the blood through the arteries—similar to the work of a faucet pumping water through a hose at high pressure. This type of hard force against the artery walls can damage them and make them susceptible to the buildup of the fatty deposits known as plaque. When plaque completely blocks the artery, and blood and oxygen can no longer flow, a heart attack may result.

Narrowed arteries, clogged with plaque, offer even less space for this high-pressure blood flow and may put up resistance against it. The heart's walls may thicken and dilate to compensate.

Pulmonary hypertension is a special form of high blood pressure that occurs in the blood vessels of the lungs. This condition is common to individuals with emphysema (see p. 127) or chronic obstructive pulmonary disease (COPD). High pressure in the lungs can lead to heart failure.

SYMPTOMS: Usually none, although you may sometimes experience a headache or shortness of breath.

A symptom of pulmonary hypertension is a swelling of the body, especially the legs and stomach.

Areas to Treat/Types of Manipulation

Work both feet completely first. Then find the locations of reflexes that correspond to these organs (see Chapter 3 for guidance):

1. Solar Plexus: With thumb tip, apply gradual pressure in the middle of the reflex, and work out to the edges.
2. Kidney/Adrenals: Use direct pressure with thumb tip on these reflexes.

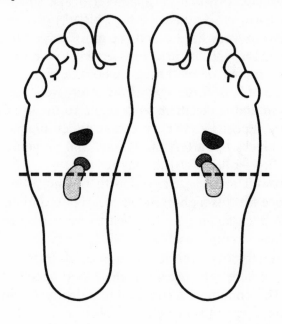

PREVENTIVE MEASURES AND COMPLEMENTARY TREATMENTS

Reflexology works well in conjunction with other alternative therapies and commonsense measures. For example:

KNOW YOUR PRESSURE: Get regular readings so that you're aware of your regular blood pressure. A normal pressure is considered to be less than 140/90.

STOP SMOKING: When you inhale cigarette tars and nicotine, you greatly restrict the amount of oxygen in your blood. By eliminating tobacco smoke from your system, your blood vessels will open up.

CHANGE YOUR LIFESTYLE: Small changes, like losing weight, getting on a regular exercise program, limiting the salt in your diet, and reducing stress can make a big difference in your blood pressure. The combination of these changes can give the heart a rest and allow blood to flow more freely through the arteries.

MEDITATE DAILY: When you quiet the mind, you also quiet the body. A daily practice of "sitting," without any particular goal or intention, can reduce both blood pressure and heart rate—both during meditation and for several hours afterward.

PRACTICE YOGA OR TAI CHI CHUAN: The gentlest postures of either of these two types of meditative exercise can calm you and teach you how to relax. By working with an experienced teacher, you will learn patience and breathing as you hold a dynamic posture or move through space.

If neither reflexology nor any of the above alternative measures have created an actual drop in your measured blood pressure and you are consistently above 140/90, consult a physician.

Hypoglycemia

It's been hours since breakfast, but you were too busy to stop for lunch. Now, suddenly, your heart is pounding in your chest, you have a throbbing headache, and you can't see straight. If you don't eat something immediately, you're going to pass out.

Hypoglycemia is a state of having extremely low blood sugar. When you consume food, your body breaks it down into its various components: amino acids from protein, glucose from carbohydrates and sugar. When you digest food, your pancreas secretes a hormone called insulin. This hormone allows the body's cells to absorb the glucose for fuel and thereby reduces sugar levels in the blood.

In fasting hypoglycemia, when you restrict food on purpose or just forget to eat, there isn't enough glucose present in the blood. This situation of course is temporary (except for heavy drinkers, whose alcohol consumption deregulates the liver's ability to store sugar) and can be remedied with a quick carbohydrate boost.

In reactive hypoglycemia, your pancreas secretes too much insulin (which in turn lowers your blood sugar too fast). This generally occurs after meals, when the body is trying to digest food, and is common in those with adult-onset diabetes and individuals who have had portions of their stomach surgically removed.

SYMPTOMS: Extreme weakness, dizziness, palpitations, nervousness, visual disturbances, confusion, and fainting.

AREAS TO TREAT/TYPES OF MANIPULATION

Work both feet completely first. Then find the locations of reflexes that correspond to these organs, and work in the following order (see Chapter 3 for guidance):

1. Pancreas: Apply direct circular pressure with thumb tip.
2. Pituitary: Apply direct pressure with thumb tip.
3. Thyroid: Work "necks" of toes with thumb tip.
4. Liver/gallbladder: Apply direct pressure to gallbladder reflex; then glide up and to left across liver.
5. Adrenals: Apply direct pressure with thumb tip.

PREVENTIVE MEASURES AND COMPLEMENTARY TREATMENTS

Reflexology works well in conjunction with other alternative therapies and commonsense measures. For example:

KEEP YOUR SUGAR UP WITH SNACKS: Many experts believe that in order to keep your blood glucose level on an even keel, it's better to eat six small meals rather than three large ones daily. If you know that you typically feel weak and dizzy when you don't eat, carry some crackers or Life Savers with you.

WATCH YOUR EXERCISE LEVELS: It's particularly important not to knock yourself out running a marathon or taking several high-impact aerobics classes in a row without supplementing your carbohydrates. Many "sports drinks" on the market are filled with nutrients to keep your blood sugar level.

EAT HIGH PROTEIN, LOW SUGAR: In general, a person prone to hypoglycemia should maintain a diet low enough in carbohydrates and sugars so that the pancreas doesn't overreact in its insulin production. This

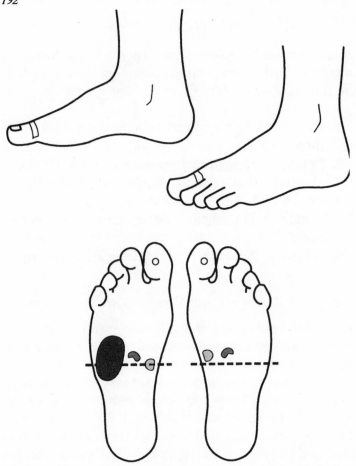

means eating more protein (well-trimmed meat and poultry, fish, legumes, and eggs), which can keep blood sugar mounting slowly in the blood rather than bumping up too quickly.

If reflexology and proper eating and exercising have not eliminated your hypoglycemic attacks, or if you black out frequently, you should see a physician for a blood test and an assessment of your pancreatic function.

Immune System Booster

You seem to get every cold and flu that comes around; you bruise easily, and you're terribly sensitive to pollen and dander. It feels as if the environment is out to get you, but what's really going on is that your internal environment isn't protecting you sufficiently.

The immune system is an interlocking group of powerful agents, including the white blood cells, their various elements, and the lymph system, that recognize foreign "invaders" and protect the body from disease. When an outside substance, an antigen such as bacteria or a virus, enters the body, the immune system goes into high gear. The lymph nodes throughout the body, as well as the bone marrow, manufacture lymphocytes, the white blood cells that filter harmful organisms out of the blood. Some of these lymphocytes call up specialized proteins, or antibodies, to fight the invader.

First, the white blood cells called T-cells recognize that something is going wrong in the system. They alert other cells—natural killer (NK) cells as well as T-cells and B-cells—which either attack the antigen directly or produce special proteins to neutralize the foreign agents.

We are born with certain types of immunity (acquired or passive immunity), and throughout our lives, as we are exposed to more viruses and bacteria, we develop additional active immunity. We may also get immunity artificially, through vaccines against certain diseases. Your immune system may flag if you are under a great deal of long-term stress or if you are in a foreign country where the foreign agents are different from those you're used to at home. Some diseases, such as lupus, certain cancers, and AIDS, can destroy the immune system of the body, as can courses of chemotherapy or radiation or exposure to hazardous waste materials in the environment or on the job.

When the immune system is lowered, you are susceptible to any illness that comes down the pike. Reflexology can help reverse the problem, however, and boost the system—whether you're already very sick or wish to use it as preventive treatment.

SYMPTOMS: If your immune system is defective, you will experience general malaise, fatigue, constant colds and flu, rashes, bruises, and hair loss. You may not be able to muster the energy to eat or exercise properly, and this may further depress your immune system.

AREAS TO TREAT/TYPES OF MANIPULATION

Work both feet completely first. Then find the locations of reflexes that correspond to these organs, and work in the following order (see Chapter 3 for guidance):

1. Lymph Glands: Work thumb tip and pad gently back and forth across area.
2. Spleen: Apply gradual circular pressure with thumb tip and pad.
3. Colon: Beginning on the right foot, apply direct pressure with your thumb tip to the ileocecal valve; then glide the thumb tip from this valve up the ascending colon, across the transverse colon, to the inside edge of the foot.

   Switch to the left foot. Glide the thumb tip left to right across the transverse colon, down the descending colon, and end with a slight hook upward at the sigmoid colon.

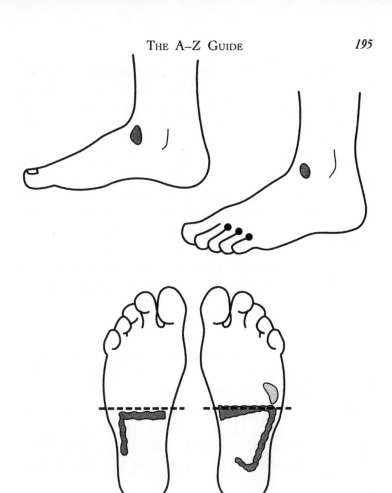

PREVENTIVE MEASURES AND COMPLEMENTARY TREATMENTS

Reflexology works well in conjunction with other alternative therapies and commonsense measures. For example:

TREAT YOURSELF WELL: Eliminate junk food and processed food, cut out cigarettes and alcohol, exercise daily, and get enough sleep. If you've been working compulsively, make an appointment with yourself for a half hour "quiet time" each day, when you can listen to music, meditate, or sit in the sun with your cat.

TRY HERBS: Various herbal tonics will stimulate the immune system. Brew an infusion of stinging nettle to nourish the adrenals (take 1 cup or more of dried leaf infusion daily). You may also take 20 drops of echinacea/goldenseal extract daily for an additional boost.

SUPPLEMENT YOUR SYSTEM: Vitamin B_6 (pyridoxine) will get your immune system in gear. You can take 50 mg. daily and eat foods containing this vitamin, such as baked potato with the skin on, broccoli, prunes, bananas, legumes, and all meats, poultry, and fish. Vitamin C (500 to 1,000 mg. daily) will help you ward off infections and heal wounds more quickly. The mineral selenium (usually packaged commercially with vitamin E) also strengthens your immune system; you can take a supplement or get it in foods such as seaweed, grains, garlic, liver, fish, and shellfish.

TRY YOGA OR TAI CHI CHUAN: Both these forms of meditative exercise (the first from India, the second from China) will improve immune function. By using the breath to stimulate various parts of the body as you hold dynamic postures and then relax completely (yoga) or as you move in a choreographed form (tai chi chuan), you can build up reserves of energy that may help you do more and feel better.

If neither reflexology nor any of the alternative therapies listed above seem to improve your fatigue and susceptibility to illness, see your physician for a thorough checkup.

Impotence
(Erectile Dysfunction)

You can't get it up. Or perhaps you can, but it doesn't stay that way. As nice as she is, as much as she protests it doesn't matter and you should relax, it's impossible: There is nothing else on your mind and nothing at all down there.

"Impotence" is the old term for what sex therapists now refer to as erectile dysfunction, which means difficulty achieving an erection and completing the act of intercourse. This problem is generally more prevalent in the older male population (about 55 percent of all men over 75 and from 10 to 20 million men of all ages have experienced erectile dysfunction at some time).

The penis is made of a spongelike tissue with many spaces where blood can flow in. In its flaccid state these spaces are relatively empty, but when a man is aroused, they fill with blood and distend, engorging the cavernous bodies of the penis and making it hard. The higher the level of erotic interest, the greater the ease of erection, although any type of physical contact or stimulation, such as a casual touch, the vibration of a car or train, or even getting the penis lodged at a certain angle inside underwear, may cause an erection. Hormonal production also plays a part; a sufficient amount of the male gonadal hormone testosterone is partly responsible for normal erectile function.

Problems that prevent erections may be physical or psychological or both. In the case of physical dysfunction, inadequate blood flow to the penis may be caused by such heart problems as atherosclerosis or hypertension, diabetes, muscular dystrophy, epilepsy, spinal cord damage, chronic pain, lung disease, alcoholism and drug abuse, or thyroid or hormonal problems. Use and abuse of medications—particularly antihypertensive medicines—may keep you from getting an erection.

When there is psychological dysfunction, lack of or inhibited desire, sexual repression, anger at your partner, boredom with an old partner, anxiety with a new partner, trying too hard to please your partner, concerns about your job or children or aging parents, financial or legal worries, or the general fatigue and stress of daily life, erectile function may be affected.

SYMPTOMS: The inability to achieve and maintain an erection sufficient for penetration and ejaculation during three out of four attempts.

AREAS TO TREAT/TYPES OF MANIPULATION

Work both feet completely first. Then find the locations of reflexes that correspond to these organs, and work in the following order (see Chapter 3 for guidance):

1. Pituitary: Apply direct pressure with thumb tip.
2. Solar Plexus: With thumb tip, apply gradual pressure in the center of the reflex, and work out to the edges.
3. Thyroid/Parathyroid: Work "necks" of toes with thumb tip.
4. Adrenals: Apply direct pressure with thumb tip.
5. Testes: Apply gradual circular pressure with thumb tip and pad.
6. Prostate: Apply gradual circular pressure with thumb tip and pad.

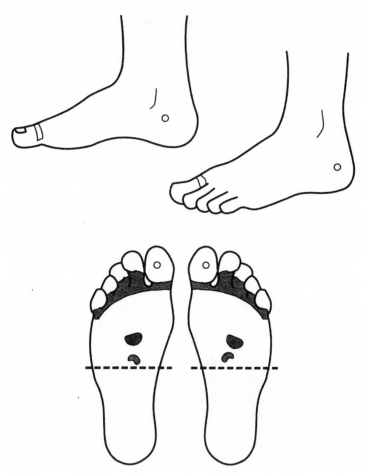

PREVENTIVE MEASURES AND COMPLEMENTARY TREATMENTS

Reflexology works well in conjunction with other alternative therapies and commonsense measures. For example:

PLAY WITH YOUR PARTNER OUT OF BED: It's a good idea to have fun together out of the sexual arena. Rake leaves, go dancing, cook a meal together, watch a sunset, or play with your dog. You'll find that the intimacy you share outside the bedroom may ease the tension inside.

PLAY WITH YOURSELF: Masturbation is a wonderful way to discover your own pleasures without the pressure of having to please a partner. You may wish to leaf through an erotic magazine or watch an erotic film as you stimulate yourself.

USE A LUBRICANT: The slippery feeling of saliva, Astroglide, Today Personal Lubricant, or any of the lubricants available in pharmacies and sex shops can heighten the sensitivity of the penis and make it more responsive to touch.

THROW AWAY YOUR CIGARETTES: Tars and nicotine reduce the amount of oxygen in your blood, making it harder for blood to travel to the extremities—hands, feet, and penis. If you are concerned about your fertility as well as your potency, it's important to know that men who smoke have lower sperm counts, less sperm motility, and more abnormal sperm than nonsmokers.

CUT DOWN ON MEDICATIONS: Your over-the-counter drugs as well as prescription medications can wreak havoc with your sex life. Tranquilizers, diuretics, antidepressants, antipsychotics, painkillers, barbiturates, and ulcer drugs, as well as antihypertensive medications like Inderal, Blocadren, Levatol, and Corgard have been shown to create erectile problems in many users.

If neither reflexology nor any of the alternative therapies listed above seem to improve your erectile function, see your physician. A specialist—a urologist or sex therapist—may be able to diagnose and treat your problem.

Incontinence

When you wet yourself for the first time sitting in the movie laughing, you thought it was just a weird accident. But these days you can't seem to hold it anytime. The idea of adult diapers has to be the worst embarrassment in the world. If only there were someone you could tell, but you can't.

More than ten million adult Americans (most of them women) are incontinent. The problem is not inevitable, and it can be controlled and in some cases reversed.

As we age, the pelvic floor muscles don't have the same elasticity they used to. This means that any increase in pressure on the abdomen (like coughing or sneezing) stresses the bladder. Another part of this problem is a decrease in blood flow in the lower urinary tract and in the number of cells in the mucous membranes of the urethra as we age. Both blood flow and mucosal cells are necessary to give sufficient pressure so that the urethra can close completely after voiding. In women the decline in estrogen after menopause accelerates these problems since the cells of the bladder and urethra depend on their estrogen receptors to help maintain function.

If you suffer from stress incontinence, you will leak a small amount of urine when the bladder is stressed through coughing, laughing, sneezing, or having an orgasm. As the urethra becomes thinner and you lose muscle tone, it's harder for the pelvic floor muscles to hold on to the urine.

If you suffer from urge incontinence, you may have an uncontrollable need to go to the bathroom even if you've just gone, or you may wet the bed at night. The cause is an inability to control the muscle that usually contracts to hold back urine but that now doesn't function properly. Other causes may be infection, inflammation, bladder stones, or stool impaction.

Mixed incontinence is the term used when both conditions occur simultaneously.

SYMPTOMS: Leaking urine when coughing, laughing, sneezing, or having an orgasm; having an overwhelming urge to urinate and not being able to hold your urine; feeling that you have to void again just after you have urinated.

AREAS TO TREAT/TYPES OF MANIPULATION

Work both feet completely first. Then find the locations of reflexes that correspond to these organs, and work in the following order (see Chapter 3 for guidance):

1. Kidneys: Apply direct pressure with thumb tip.
2. Adrenals: Apply direct pressure with thumb tip.
3. Ureter: Glide thumb tip down ureter from kidney to bladder.
4. Bladder: Apply circular pressure with thumb pad.

PREVENTIVE MEASURES AND COMPLEMENTARY TREATMENTS

Reflexology works well in conjunction with other alternative therapies and commonsense measures. For example:

DON'T HIDE THE PROBLEM: Hidden incontinence can lead to a life spent stuck at home for fear of having an accident. It's important to share this information with your general practitioner or gynecologist. She or he will help you to manage this condition with natural or conventional medical treatments.

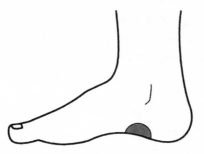

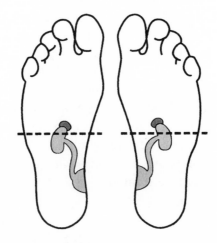

GET ON SCHEDULE: One of the most helpful treatments are bladder drills, in which you ingest a certain amount of fluid and void at regular intervals. You may start out with half-hour drills (even if you think you don't have to go this frequently), and work your way up to two or three hours.

DO YOUR KEGELS: These exercises improve the tone of muscles around the pelvic floor. In order to do one Kegel, imagine that you are sitting on the toilet releasing the flow of urine. Now contract the muscles around the urethra, stopping the flow. You should practice three sets of ten three times daily. Do them slowly, quickly, holding the contraction, then letting it go.

DON'T TAKE DRINKS THAT STIMULATE THE BLADDER: Alcohol, caffeine, grapefruit juice, and sodas all tend to have a diuretic effect. Try substituting other drinks and see if your condition improves.

TAKE AN HERBAL BREAK: To strengthen the bladder, take a cup of dried teasel root (1 tablespoon to a cup of water boiled for ten minutes).

To prevent urge incontinence, try 10 to 20 drops of black cohosh tincture once or twice a day for several weeks or as needed. (IF YOU ARE PREGNANT, YOU SHOULD NOT USE THIS HERB UNTIL THE LAST TRIMESTER.) Other helpful antispasmodic herbs are ginger, catnip, and cornsilk; take a cup of any one of these daily.

If neither reflexology nor any of the alternative therapies listed above seem to improve your ability to hold your urine, see your physician. Incontinence can be a symptom that indicates you have an infection or inflammation or some obstruction in the bladder or urethra that should be treated.

INDIGESTION (SEE ALSO HEARTBURN, P. 166)

"I can't believe I ate the whole thing," ran the copy of a popular commercial that illustrated the problem of indigestion. And it's true: You didn't think; you just ate. And ate and ate. All that fried, fatty food and a big shake to wash it down. Now you're paying for it: the queasiness, the bloated feeling. You just wish they'd go away.

If you have indigestion, also known as dyspepsia, you have a flaw in the digestive process. This is usually due to overeating or excessive drinking, or both, which causes an inflammation of the stomach lining. Smoking can contribute to this problem.

Ulcers can cause indigestion, as can gallstones (see p. 146) and hiatal hernias (see p. 180). But perhaps the most flagrant instigator of indigestion is stress: a family dispute that carries over to the dinner table; a tense meeting with the boss over lunch; dinner with an elderly parent fraught with criticism and complaints.

For most people, indigestion is a temporary problem, generally solved by changing eating habits, lowering stress, and making the experience of eating more leisurely and comfortable.

SYMPTOMS: Pain, heartburn, belching, flatulence, nausea, and full feeling in the abdomen.

AREAS TO TREAT/TYPES OF MANIPULATION

Work both feet completely first. Then find the locations of reflexes that correspond to these organs, and work in the following order (see Chapter 3 for guidance):

1. Stomach: Apply gradual circular pressure with thumb tip and pad.
2. Solar Plexus: With thumb tip, apply gradual pressure in the center of the reflex, and work out to the edges.
3. Colon: Beginning on the right foot, apply direct pressure with your thumb tip to the ileocecal valve; then glide the thumb tip from this valve up the

ascending colon, across the transverse colon, to the inside edge of the foot.

Switch to the left foot. Glide the thumb tip left to right across the transverse colon, down the descending colon, and end with a slight hook upward at the sigmoid colon.

4. Small Intestine: Glide thumb back and forth and up and down through area.

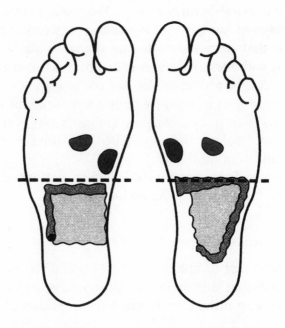

Preventive Measures and Complementary Treatments

Reflexology works well in conjunction with other alternative therapies and commonsense measures. For example:

DON'T OVERDO: Your stomach has stretch receptors that allow it to accept more food than your brain actually wants to assuage the hunger you feel. It takes about fifteen minutes for your brain to catch up with your stomach. So eat half of what you think you want, and take a break. If you're still hungry after a quarter of an hour, eat some more.

SIT DOWN AND RELAX: The slower you eat, the better for your digestion. The more comfortable you are as you consume your food, the better you can process it. So try changing old habits, like eating standing up, walking around, slumped in a couch in front of the TV, or in the car.

VISUALIZE YOUR FOOD: Before you eat, think about the process of eating. Imagine the food on your plate, and be grateful that it's waiting for you. Spend some time thinking about what it will taste like in your mouth, how swallowing will feel, and then how your stomach will accept what you've consumed and break it down into its usable parts to nourish and support your body. As you do this exercise, make it a very sensual experience: Smell and taste and see your food clearly before you think about eating. This mind game is practice for the same exercise you will eventually do as you sit down at the table.

If neither reflexology nor any of the alternative therapies listed above seem to improve your digestion, see your physician.

INFECTION

The sore on your elbow won't heal; instead it's hot, red, and tender to the touch. Actually your whole body feels sore, as though it were fighting off a foreign enemy that has taken up residence in your arm.

An infection is the sign that bacteria, a virus, a fungus, or protozoa have threatened your body's well-being. As various microorganisms (antigens) break through the barrier of skin or mucous membranes, they create colonies in the bloodstream or on the inner surface of an organ. During the incubation period this colony multiplies, and the area becomes inflamed from the various toxins released by bacteria at the site of infection and as a result of the immune system's battle with the invader. As specialized white blood cells (antibodies) go to work to knock out the foreign agent and get rid of the infection it has caused, fever often results.

An animal bite can bring on an infection, as can a blister, a boil, a toothache, or an abundance of yeast in your urinary tract. You may have a local infection, for example, at the site of a wound that's gotten some dirt in it or a general infection, which can be as contagious as a common cold.

SYMPTOMS: Pain, redness, heat, or swelling around a wound or sore area; fever; general malaise.

AREAS TO TREAT/TYPES OF MANIPULATION

Work both feet completely first. Then find the locations of reflexes that correspond to these organs, and work in the following order (see Chapter 3 for guidance):

1. Lymph Glands: Work thumb tip and pad gently back and forth across area.
2. Spleen: Apply gradual circular pressure with thumb tip and pad.
3. Kidneys: Apply direct pressure with thumb tip.
4. Adrenals: Apply direct pressure with thumb tip.
5. Work reflex corresponding to affected area of body.

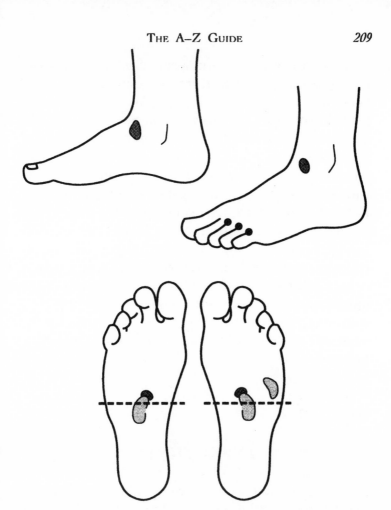

PREVENTIVE MEASURES AND COMPLEMENTARY TREATMENTS

Reflexology works well in conjunction with other alternative therapies and commonsense measures. For example:

KEEP THE WOUND CLEAN AND COVERED: Any injury should be washed with hot water and soap, dabbed with a disinfectant, and covered with a bandage. Changing the dressing regularly will keep it clean and also give you an opportunity to check for signs of infection.

STAY IN BED AND REST: Any general infection tends to make you feel awful and feverish. Running around and continuing with your regular schedule will only make you feel worse. Be kind to yourself. Sleep off the fever and dose yourself with two aspirin or Tylenol every four to six hours.

USE ICE, NOT HEAT: It's best to keep the area cold, even if heat feels better. If you've got a toothache, for example, putting warm washcloths on your face may spread the infection to the outside of the jaw.

Reflexology and alternative treatments will usually help reduce an infection and speed healing. However, if you are still running a fever and the infected site is red and angry-looking after three days, consult a physician. Infections may run their course, but they can also become serious enough to require antibiotic treatment.

INFERTILITY

You've been trying to conceive a child for a year, and you're beginning to wonder if it's just fate. Unprotected sex always got people pregnant in high school, so what's going on? Even your good relationship feels strained when you step into the bedroom.

Infertility is a temporary inability to conceive a child. It is a treatable condition, unlike sterility, which is a permanent condition. In one third of all cases the problem lies with the woman, in another third the problem lies with the man, and in the remaining third both partners have some problem. A woman's fertility naturally declines with age after thirty-one; a man's fertility begins to decline after forty. Therefore, for many two-career couples who are beginning to try when they're beyond their peak fertility years, the prospects seem daunting.

Major causes of male infertility are a sperm count of less than twenty million (reasons might be low testosterone levels, exposure to hazardous chemicals or radiation, heat, or too frequent sexual activity), low sperm motility (sperm that move so slowly they can't reach the egg in time to fertilize it), or abnormally shaped sperm. Other problems are obstructions in the tubes that carry the sperm from the testes, varicose veins in the scrotum, or retrograde ejaculation, in which the semen moves back into the bladder instead of being propelled into the vagina (this condition may be caused by prostate problems or use of antihypertensive medication).

Major causes of female infertility are not ovulating, a short luteal phase (the second half of the menstrual cycle after ovulation), an endocrine problem that affects estrogen and progesterone production or other hormones produced by the pituitary or thyroid glands, endometriosis (a disease in which tissue from the uterine lining lodges elsewhere in the body), blocked fallopian tubes (which prevent the egg from traveling from the ovaries to the uterus), and an infection or a sexually transmitted disease that has irritated the tubes or formed scar tissue in the area.

The couple together may have an acid/alkaline imbalance—that is, her cervical secretions may kill off his sperm before they can ever reach the egg. Another dual problem is stress; feelings of tension can alter the hormonal environment in the uterus and make it hostile to the creation of new life.

Many of these problems can be addressed and solved over time, as long as the couple is patient and is willing to try a variety of options.

SYMPTOMS: The inability of a couple to conceive a child after one year of unprotected sex.

Areas to Treat/Types of Manipulation

Both partners should do a treatment. Work both feet completely first. Then find the locations of reflexes that correspond to these organs, and work in the following order (see Chapter 3 for guidance):

1. Testes/Ovaries: Apply gradual circular pressure with thumb tip and pad.
2. Prostate/Uterus: Apply gradual circular pressure with thumb tip and pad.
3. Pituitary: Apply direct pressure with thumb tip.

Preventive Measures and Complementary Treatments

Reflexology works well in conjunction with other alternative therapies and commonsense measures. For example:

CHART YOUR TEMPERATURE AND MUCUS: A temperature chart will tell you the day you ovulate (your temperature suddenly rises); a check of your cervical mucus will alert you to fertile days. The mucus will be wet and slippery and form a thread between two fingers on fertile days right before ovulation (before your temperature rises) and three days after; it will then change to a thick, creamy consistency; and finally, on nonfertile days, it will be crumbly and dry.

CONTROL YOUR STRESS: Some type of daily relaxation technique (meditation, visualization, yoga, tai chi chuan, and so forth) will put you on the right path to achieving your goal. You will find, as your body, mind, and spirit learn to relax, that your attitude toward conception will become less frenzied and more focused.

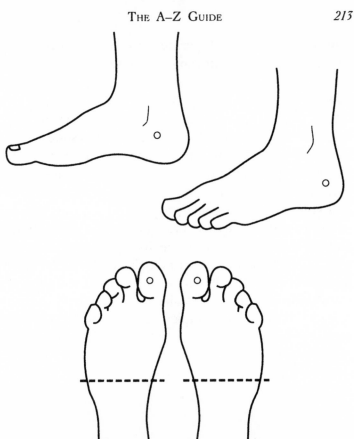

ENJOY MASSAGE TOGETHER: Touch can be an important tool in communication between couples and may revitalize a relationship that is burned out from intercourse solely for the sake of conception. At least once a week give each other a full body massage. You can use aromatherapy oils such as neroli, rose, and jasmine for the woman, and sandalwood, frankincense, and patchouli for the man.

USE NATURAL LUBRICATION: Commercial lubricants can cut down on sperm motility and survival, so use your own saliva or room-temperature egg whites or plain yogurt to get moisture flowing during sex.

STAY WHERE YOU ARE AFTER SEX: Make sure you have enough time after making love to stay in bed and give the sperm the best chance of swimming upstream. The woman can put her legs up on her partner's shoulders or the headboard for about half an hour after sex. This also gives the couple time together to lie still and enjoy each other's company.

If you have not become pregnant within one year (or several months longer if the woman is over thirty-five and the man is over fifty), see your physician. You may wish to consult an endocrinologist who specializes in infertility, and after having a full medical workup, you can decide whether you wish to continue with reflexology and alternative therapies or to try medical/surgical care.

INFLUENZA

If someone could just put you out of your misery, you would be eternally grateful. Your head pounds; your whole body aches; your stomach is a mess; you have a fever that seems to get higher by the hour. On top of everything else, you feel weak as a kitten, and it's hard to breathe.

The flu comes to most of us at least once a season, usually during the winter, when several strains of virus are rampant. The Asian flu (the most serious strain) is an A type of virus, whereas the B and C types cause only mild illnesses. These three types may mutate into so many different forms that you can easily contract another flu quickly after recovering from the first bout.

Flu vaccines can be protective, so that even if you contract the illness, you will get a milder case of it. Doctors generally recommend that individuals at high risk, particularly those over sixty-five, get flu shots every October.

Flu is contagious, so it tends to pass from family member to family member through sputum, saliva, and droplets from an infected person's sneezes and coughs. The incubation period is generally a day or two, after which the illness hits full force and may last several days to a week.

It is vital to stay in bed and let the flu run its course. If you don't, you risk another infection on top of it, such as bronchitis or pneumonia. In very young children and the elderly, this situation can be fatal.

SYMPTOMS: Headache, muscle and joint ache, fever, extreme fatigue, general malaise, nausea, diarrhea, lack of appetite. Depending on the strain, you may also have such upper respiratory symptoms as coughing, sneezing, and sinus congestion.

AREAS TO TREAT/TYPES OF MANIPULATION

Work both feet completely first. Then find the locations of reflexes that correspond to these organs, and work in the following order (see Chapter 3 for guidance):

1. Sinus: Using thumb tip, first work tips of toes, using circular motion; then work all around the whole toe.
2. Lungs: With tip and edge of thumb, work up and down and left to right.
3. Bronchi: With tip and edge of both thumbs, glide from the bases of the toes down toward the instep.

4. Lymph Glands: Work thumb tip and pad gently back and forth across area.
5. Spleen: Apply circular pressure with thumb tip and pad.
6. Kidneys: Apply direct pressure with thumb tip.
7. Adrenals: Apply direct pressure with thumb tip.

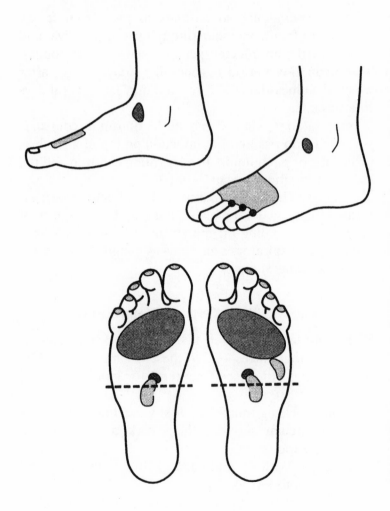

Preventive Measures and Complementary Treatments

Reflexology works well in conjunction with other alternative therapies and commonsense measures. For example:

TAKE CARE OF YOURSELF: Stay in bed and keep warm. Try to avoid drafts so you won't get chilled. Get a lot of sleep (you probably won't be able to keep your eyes open), and listen to music or books on tape when you're up.

DRINK TO YOUR FLU'S DISCONTENT: Fluids will provide the nutrients you need, especially if you're too queasy to eat. They will also keep you from getting dehydrated. Stay away from caffeinated beverages and sodas; drink lots of hot herbal teas, pure springwater, and fruit juices.

STAY AWAY FROM YOUR LOVED ONES: Flu is contagious, so if you can, sleep by yourself, avoid kissing and hugging your loved ones, and if you absolutely have to go out to get food or provisions, keep a scarf over your nose and mouth.

TAKE ASPIRIN FOR FEVER AND ACHES: Two aspirin every four hours (Tylenol only for children) will reduce fever and take away some of your achiness.

Influenza can be very serious—even life-threatening—in the elderly and the very young. If neither reflexology nor any of the alternative therapies listed have improved your symptoms, or if you have chest pain or difficulty breathing or are bringing up yellowish-green phlegm, see your physician.

✳

KIDNEY STONES

There's a sudden searing pain around your waist. Suddenly you're fine. Then the pain comes again, worse than anything you've ever experienced. It hurts to urinate, and when you do, the stream is tinged with blood.

Kidney stones are mineral (usually calcium) deposits that harden into masses in the urinary tract or kidney. A common condition that encourages the growth of stones is gout (see p. 151), in which the body is unable to get rid of sufficient uric acid, which crystallizes into stones. The same may occur with blockages in the urinary tract. Retaining urine leads to a concentration of waste products that then develop into hardened masses. Individuals who consume a great deal of milk and dairy foods and a lot of vitamin D may also be at higher risk for kidney stones, which may form when there is more calcium in the urine than the body can process. Broken bones also put you at higher risk; calcium from the fracture may leach into the urine, where it forms stones.

If the stones move so that they block or press against a portion of the kidney, they can cause extreme pain, as can the act of passing the stone through the urethra.

If you've passed one stone, it's likely you will develop others. A change of lifestyle along with your reflexology treatments may make the next smaller and easier to pass, however.

SYMPTOMS: There may be no symptoms until a stone becomes lodged in the urethra and cannot pass. Individuals who do have symptoms may experience severe pain and tenderness around the kidney (just above the waist), frequent and painful urination, blood in the urine, fever, chills, and great fatigue.

AREAS TO TREAT/TYPES OF MANIPULATION

Work both feet completely first. Then find the locations of reflexes that correspond to these organs, and work in the following order (see Chapter 3 for guidance):

1. Kidneys: Apply direct pressure with thumb tip.
2. Ureter: Glide thumb tip down ureter from kidney to bladder.
3. Bladder: Apply circular pressure with thumb pad.

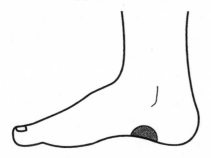

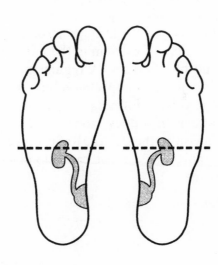

Preventive Measures and Complementary Treatments

Reflexology works well in conjunction with other alternative therapies and commonsense measures. For example:

WATCH YOUR DAIRY FOODS: If you drink three glasses of milk daily, you should cut down on yogurt, cheese, and ice cream. Although women past menopause require calcium supplements, most others should limit their intakes of both dietary and supplemental calcium and vitamin D.

DRINK WATER: If you've passed a stone, you need to dilute your urine and keep it from collecting salts and minerals that can form into new stones. Doctors recommend two quarts of pure springwater a day, more if you're exercising a lot or live in a hot climate where you sweat freely.

EAT LOW PROTEIN, LOW SALT: Protein breaks down into amino acids, which tend to increase the amount of calcium and uric acid in the urine. It's better to eat a high-carbohydrate, low-fat, and low-protein diet (the proportion should be 60:20:20). Salt, like any other mineral, can crystallize into stones. Limit your intake to two or three grams daily.

GET OUT AND EXERCISE: Both aerobic and anaerobic activity help deposit calcium in the bones instead of in the urine and bloodstream. A regular program of walking, biking, rowing, low-impact aerobics, or step training can keep stones from forming.

An attack of kidney stones or blood in your urine means a visit to the doctor. Reflexology and the alternative therapies listed above can help in a total program of wellness care.

KNEE PROBLEMS

It's not just downhill skiing that gets you; ordinary walking is painful. Maybe you twisted your knee, or put too much weight on it, or something. But it's really bad, and you have no idea what to do about it.

The knee is a combination joint—part hinge, part rotation. Its unfortunate position in the leg puts a great deal of stress on it most of the time, and exercise or unthinking movements can do damage to the muscles, ligaments, tendons, and cartilage of which it's made.

The shinbone and thighbone meet at the knee, forming a connection similar to two ball and socket joints side by side. As the bones come together, they are rimmed with cartilage (the meniscus) that keeps the joints from moving from side to side. In addition, there are seven ligaments around the knee; five surround the joint on the outside, and two cross behind the knee. There's also a tendon that starts at the quadriceps in the thigh, crosses at the kneecap, and reattaches at the shinbone. So there are many overlapping factors that contribute to the knee's stability—and to its liability.

Sports injuries are the greatest source of damage. The cartilage in the knee may tear because of a fall, a blow, or a severe twist. Since there's very little blood supply to the cartilage here, this condition heals poorly. Ligaments can also be torn at the knee because they don't have much give. Arthritis may cause pain and stiffness, and this may compound injuries or prior damage to the knee. Surgical repair is generally advised for athletes and those who demand active lives; for others, reflexology and commonsense practices may alleviate the most uncomfortable symptoms.

SYMPTOMS: Pain, stiffness, partial or total loss of flexibility and movement.

AREAS TO TREAT/TYPES OF MANIPULATION

Work both feet completely first. Then find the locations of reflexes that correspond to these organs and work in the following order (see Chapter 3 for guidance):

1. Knee: Work the end of the thumb all around the fifth metatarsal bone on the outside of each foot.
2. Shoulder: Apply firm circular pressure with thumb tip.
3. Hip: Work thumb edge all around lower edge of outer anklebone.

PREVENTIVE MEASURES AND COMPLEMENTARY TREATMENTS

Reflexology works well in conjunction with other alternative therapies and commonsense measures. For example:

LOSE WEIGHT: The less poundage the knee joint has to bear, the happier it will be. If you are more than 10 percent over your ideal weight range as determined by life insurance tables, you should get on a sensible eating program and reduce the burden on your knees.

TRY R.I.C.E.: If you've just injured your knee, or if you are in chronic pain, it's important to use rest, ice, compression, and elevation. You can wrap the knee in an Ace bandage and put an ice pack (ice plus cold water, to make it colder longer) on the propped-up knee every few hours for half an hour. While you're recuperating, take a rest from your regular schedule.

USE NSAIDS: Ibuprofen (two tablets every four hours)

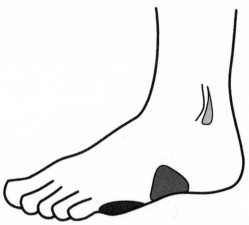

will take the edge off the pain. Studies have shown that it also improves joint mobility in people with ligament damage.

EXERCISE PREVENTIVELY: The best care is preventive, so if you're a physically active person or if you've had an injury that's healed, you ought to be doing leg lifts (as you sit against the wall with your legs out in front of you) and isometric knee contractions (open and close the joint while holding a rolled towel under the knee). You should also stretch for ten minutes before you go out to exercise, whether you're jogging, biking, or doing martial arts.

If reflexology and the alternative therapies listed above have not improved the pain or function of your knee within a month, consult your physician.

✳

MENSTRUAL CRAMPS

It's that time of the month. You don't have to look at a calendar; you know by the full, achy feeling in your ovaries, the bloating, nausea, and fatigue. They are regular reminders that you are most emphatically a woman in her reproductive years.

Menstrual cramps (or dysmenorrhea) are thought to be caused by prostaglandins, fatty acid derivatives released from the lining of the uterus just before a menstrual period begins. These substances stimulate small contractions, which tighten uterine blood vessels, causing pain. Other possible reasons for painful periods are previous severe pelvic infection or a uterus that tips backward toward the rectum.

Menstrual cramps may be a constant companion from a girl's first period in adolescence up to menopause. Or they may develop later in life, for a variety of reasons, such as fibroid tumors, endometriosis, or a narrow cervix. The range of experience is probably as wide as the number of women who menstruate: Some find cramps mildly annoying; others find them so debilitating they retreat to their beds for several days.

SYMPTOMS: Cramping or pain in the pelvis, sometimes radiating around to the lower back. This feeling may be accompanied by nausea, vomiting, diarrhea, headache, general malaise, and moodiness.

AREAS TO TREAT/TYPES OF MANIPULATION

Work both feet completely first. Then find the locations of reflexes that correspond to these organs, and work in the following order (see Chapter 3 for guidance):

1. Uterus: Apply gradual circular pressure with thumb tip and pad.
2. Ovaries: Apply gradual circular pressure with thumb tip and pad.
3. Fallopian Tubes: Glide thumb tip back and forth across area.
4. Solar Plexus: With thumb tip, apply gradual pressure in the middle of reflex, and work out to the edges.

PREVENTIVE MEASURES AND COMPLEMENTARY TREATMENTS

Reflexology works well in conjunction with other alternative therapies and commonsense measures. For example:

WARM THE AREA: Keeping a hot-water bottle or heating pad on your abdomen may alleviate the discomfort.

TAKE CALCIUM AND MAGNESIUM: These minerals not only strengthen the bones but also help the blood coagulate properly and maintain the sympathetic nervous system in proper balance. Take 800 to 1,000 mg. of calcium daily with 400 to 500 mg. of magnesium.

SHAKE UP THE AREA: Try increasing circulation in the area by doing your own form of belly dancing. Stand with your feet apart, and quickly tilt your pelvis upward, contracting the muscles around your vagina and anus. Release, and tilt backward. Contract the muscles again. Release, and tilt side to side.

MAKE LOVE: When you are sexually aroused, you get a lot of blood flow to the pelvic area, which can alleviate

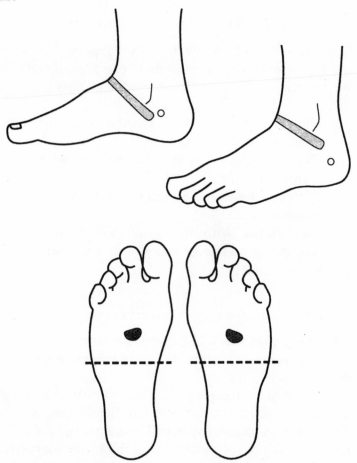

congestion. The physical release of orgasm also defeats the painful uterine contractions stimulated by the action of the prostaglandins.

TRY AN HERBAL COCKTAIL: Try analgesic herbs that will reduce or eliminate painful periods: either yarrow or black cohosh tea (3 cups daily) or 20 drops of angelica tincture before meals or 10 drops of chamomile tincture twice daily.

NO MORE CAFFEINE: Caffeine is a stimulant and irritates the tissues. If you slowly eliminate coffee, tea, chocolate, and sodas from your diet, you may see a decrease in your monthly pain.

If reflexology and the alternative therapies listed above have not improved your condition within three months, or if your pain is increasing with each cycle, consult your physician.

✳

MENOPAUSAL PROBLEMS

Sitting in a meeting at work, you are suddenly drenched with sweat. Your heart pounds away, and you feel so exhausted you want to sleep for a week, but suddenly insomnia has become a problem. Then, too, sex just doesn't feel good anymore. Is this the change of life?

Menopause, the cessation of menses, occurs somewhere between the ages of forty and fifty-eight to all women. As the ovaries stop responding to messages from the pituitary gland in the brain, the level of the hormone estrogen declines, resulting in a variety of changes in all organ systems. Cholesterol levels and blood pressure increase; bone density and mass decrease. These natural changes may also trigger certain markers of menopause. The traditional hot flash and vaginal dryness occur to many, but not all, women.

The most important considerations at this time of life are preventive care of the bones and heart since the depletion of estrogen adversely affects both. This is a time of life to revamp diet, exercise, and attitude to ensure a healthy midlife.

MARKERS: Hot flashes and night sweats, vaginal dryness, palpitations, joint pain, dizziness, ringing in the ears, weight gain and shift, short-term memory loss, formication (crawling skin), incontinence, shortness of breath, headaches, cold extremities, mouth sensitivity, dry eyes, and great fatigue.

In addition, there is a decrease in bone mass and density, as well as higher LDL ("bad") cholesterol and lower HDL ("good") cholesterol.

AREAS TO TREAT/TYPES OF MANIPULATION

Work both feet completely first. Then find the locations of reflexes that correspond to these organs, and work in the following order (see Chapter 3 for guidance):

1. Uterus: Apply gradual circular pressure with thumb tip and pad.
2. Ovaries: Apply gradual circular pressure with thumb tip and pad.
3. Endocrine System (Adrenals, Thyroid/Parathyroid, Pituitary)
   Adrenals: Apply direct pressure with thumb tip.
   Thyroid/Parathyroid: Work "necks" of toes with thumb tip.
   Pituitary: Apply direct pressure with thumb tip.

PREVENTIVE MEASURES AND COMPLEMENTARY TREATMENTS

Reflexology works well in conjunction with other alternative therapies and commonsense measures. For example:

EXERCISE: Get out every day, and walk, jog, ride a bike, swim, row, or take a dance, yoga, or martial arts class (hard-style martial arts, such as karate or judo, or soft-style, such as tai chi chuan or aikido). Studies show that daily exercise alleviates menopausal problems, increases

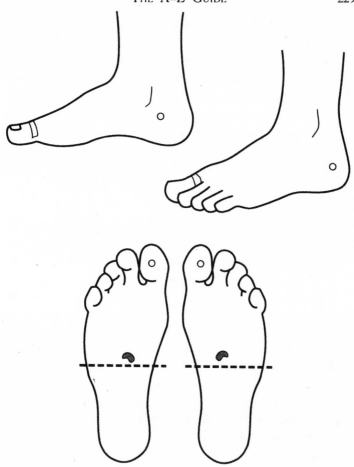

circulation and respiration, and also triggers the release of beta-endorphins, the natural opiates in the brain that give us a feeling of well-being. As we feel better psychologically, we are better able to withstand minor physical discomfort.

DRESS IN LAYERS: When you're having hot flashes, you can take off your jacket or sweater; when your body counters the flashes by chilling off, you can replace your outer garments. It's also better to wear natural fabrics—cotton, silk, wool—or those materials created for exercise, such as Capilene and polypropylene, that wick sweat away from the body.

USE LUBRICATION: In order to keep your sex life in good shape, get a water-based lubricant, and use it every time you have sex. A dab of Replens, Astroglide, or Today Personal Lubricant can make intimacy more fun and recapture the sense of comfort you used to have when aroused. If you run out of the store-bought variety, remember that saliva is the original lubricant and works perfectly well.

CHANGE YOUR EATING AND DRINKING: Six small meals instead of three large ones will allow your body's temperature to stay on an even keel. You may also wish to try cutting out caffeine (a stimulant and temperature raiser), as well as limiting alcohol and increasing your fluid intake (8 to 10 glasses of water, juice, or herbal teas daily).

HERBS TO THE RESCUE: For hot flashes, try herbs that cool your system (chickweed or elder), nourish the liver (dandelion or yellow dock), and provide natural estrogens (black cohosh or gotu kola tea). Blend these herbs for a daily cup of tea.

For excessive bleeding, try dong quai or horsetail tea. You can also eat estrogenic foods; soy is a great source, and you can find tofu, tempeh, miso, and soybeans in both Asian and general supermarkets. Essential fatty acids (EFAs) are also recommended for flooding: Take 1 to 2 tablespoons daily of evening primrose oil, flaxseed, borage, or black currant seed oil.

If reflexology and the alternative therapies listed above have not improved your condition within three months, or if you are bleeding heavily during or between cycles, consult your physician. You may wish to consider hormone replacement therapy to protect your heart and bones and to ease your passage through menopause.

NAUSEA

It comes on suddenly, and you feel bile rising in your throat. Was it something you ate, that bumpy bus ride, the fight with your boss, too much alcohol the previous night, or just the sight of someone else throwing up? It's as though your stomach had turned inside out, and you feel as if you want to die or at the very least get to a toilet FAST.

Nausea is a symptom of many physical and emotional conditions, involving an upset of the gastrointestinal system that results in a set of unpleasant sensations that may lead to throwing up. The sensation of nausea is partly triggered by the vomiting center in the brain's medulla and partly by a lot of action in the stomach and lower esophagus area.

Nausea in early pregnancy is triggered by a rapid increase in hormonal production and appears to be nature's way of forcing the new mother to eat bland and nontoxic foods to protect the growing embryo. Nibbling on crackers throughout the morning (when nausea is most common) seems to take care of the problem for most women.

Many children are prone to psychogenically induced nausea that may center on school or test anxiety or a reluctance to do certain activities the parents have been eager for them to accomplish. Adolescent girls with eating disorders also frequently feel nauseated just by looking at food.

SYMPTOMS: Queasiness, belching, retching, bringing up bile preparatory to vomiting.

Areas to Treat/Types of Manipulation

Work both feet completely first. Then find the locations of reflexes that correspond to these organs, and work in the following order (see Chapter 3 for guidance):

1. Stomach: Apply gradual circular pressure with thumb tip and pad.
2. Solar Plexus: With thumb tip, apply gradual pressure in the middle of reflex, and work out to the edges.

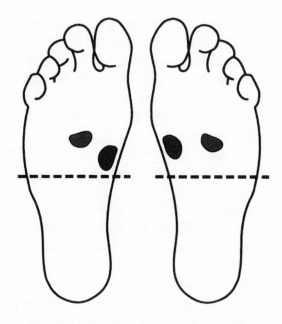

Preventive Measures and Complementary Treatments

Reflexology works well in conjunction with other alternative therapies and commonsense measures. For example:

BREATHE DEEPLY: When you think you're about to

throw up, you generally take shallow breaths. By inhaling deeply, you expand the diaphragm and alleviate the queasy sensations. Also, when you're focused on your breath, it's harder to think about the nausea.

TRY FLAT GINGER: Pop open a ginger ale, leave it out of the refrigerator, and drink it warm and flat. The concentrated carbohydrates in the soda, as well as the ginger, which is an antinausea herb, will make you feel better. You can also take a cup of ginger tea or a few capsules of powdered ginger.

PRESS YOUR POINTS: The acupuncture points for curing nausea are in the center of the webbing between your thumb and index finger. Alternating your hands, press and massage these points for five minutes on a side.

IF YOU HAVE TO, THROW UP: Nothing makes nausea feel better than allowing yourself to vomit. Although it's not a pleasant experience, it clears out the stomach acids that have been riling up your gastrointestinal system and making you feel miserable.

If reflexology and the alternative therapies listed above do not take the edge off your nausea, and you are losing a significant amount of weight, consult your physician. You may also wish to take a home pregnancy test, if you are female, to see if your symptoms are really part of your first-trimester adjustment.

Phlebitis (Thrombophlebitis)

You can't walk for the pain. The blood vessels in your legs are inflamed and swollen, and you can't tell whether it's just the superficial ones in the top layers of your skin or whether you may have the deep vein variety, which could be fatal.

Phlebitis is most commonly a simple inflammation of the superficial blood vessels, or it can be deep vein thrombophlebitis, which may trigger a blood clot that moves throughout the system and lodges in the lung. (The prefix "thrombo" refers to blood clots.)

Individuals who smoke, abuse alcohol, don't get enough exercise, and have poor circulation are at high risk for this condition. Just staying still, being confined to your bed after surgery, taking a long airplane ride or a car trip, may also cause the blood to pool in the veins. Once you've had phlebitis, it is likely to recur.

Areas to Treat/Types of Manipulation

Work both feet completely first. Then find the locations of reflexes that correspond to these organs, and work in the following order (see Chapter 3 for guidance):

1. Liver/gallbladder: Apply direct pressure with thumb tip to gallbladder; then glide up and to left across liver.
2. Adrenals: Apply direct pressure with thumb tip.

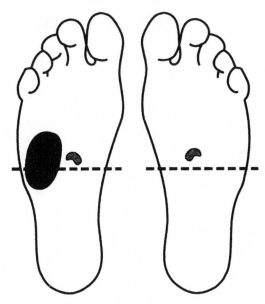

PREVENTIVE MEASURES AND COMPLEMENTARY TREATMENTS

Reflexology works well in conjunction with other alternative therapies and commonsense measures. For example:

GO OUT FOR A WALK: It's important to keep your circulation active so that the veins (a low-pressure system) can work properly. When you walk, ride a bike, or do any activity in which you use your legs, you keep the blood from flowing backward and pooling in the veins.

GET OFF THE PILL: It has been shown that oral contraceptives greatly increase your risk of deep vein clotting. If you have a history of phlebitis or any other clotting problem, you should speak to your physician about getting off the pill and on a diaphragm.

KEEP YOUR FEET ELEVATED: Blood can flow through the veins more freely when you don't have the weight of gravity pulling it down. If you're taking a break during the day, and even at night when you sleep, prop your feet up.

WEAR SUPPORT STOCKINGS: Although support won't do much to heal the condition, by keeping pressure on the veins, it alleviates discomfort in most individuals. Try these stockings and see if you like them.

You should be under a doctor's care if you have phlebitis. Reflexology and the alternative therapies listed above can help increase circulation and balance your venous system.

PNEUMONIA

It was just a cold at first, but it hung on and on. Your cough sounds like something out of a jungle film, and your chest feels raw and chafed inside. All you want to do is sleep.

Pneumonia is a lung infection in which the sacs that hold oxygen become inflamed and filled with fluid and white blood cells as they try to fight off the infection, which may be caused by a virus, bacteria, a fungus, or some other microorganism.

With lobar pneumonia, only one lobe of a lung is involved; with double pneumonia, all or parts of both lungs are involved. Bronchial pneumonia affects the upper areas of the lungs near the bronchi that connect the windpipe and lungs; walking pneumonia is a less severe form of the infection, with only a cough as a sign that something is wrong.

Pneumonia is often a secondary infection that sets in after a bad cold, flu, or case of bronchitis has lowered resistance and the body is unable to fight the new foreign invader. It may also come on as a result of diseases like emphysema, asthma, diabetes, cancer, or sickle-cell anemia. An elderly person who has fallen and broken bones and is consequently bedridden may come down with a serious pneumonia as a result of lying prone with a lowered immune system for weeks on end.

SYMPTOMS: The classic symptoms are chest pain, a sudden rise in temperature, a barking cough, and difficulty breathing. Additional symptoms of bacterial pneumonia are chills, high fever, shallow breathing, and production of dark yellow or rust-colored sputum. Additional symptoms of viral pneumonia are cold symptoms and fatigue. With either variety, you may also experience headache, nausea, and vomiting, and as your lungs can't get enough oxygen, your lips and fingertips may turn blue.

AREAS TO TREAT/TYPES OF MANIPULATION

Work both feet completely first. Then find the locations of reflexes that correspond to these organs, and work in the following order (see Chapter 3 for guidance):

1. Sinus: Using thumb tip, first work tips of toes, using circular motion; then work all around the whole toe.
2. Lungs: With tip and edge of thumb, work up and down and left to right.
3. Bronchi: With tip and edge of both thumbs, glide from the bases of the toes down toward the instep.
4. Ileocecal Valve: Apply direct pressure with thumb tip.
5. Colon: Beginning on the right foot, glide the thumb tip from the ileocecal valve up the ascending colon, across the transverse colon, to the inside edge of the foot.

Continue with the left foot. Glide the thumb left to right across the transverse colon, down the descending colon, and end with a slight hook upward at the sigmoid colon.

6. Lymph Glands: Work thumb pad and tip gently back and forth across area.
7. Spleen: Apply gradual circular pressure with thumb tip and pad.

Preventive Measures and Complementary Treatments

Reflexology works well in conjunction with other alternative therapies and commonsense measures. For example:

TAKE CARE OF YOUR COLDS: If you have symptoms (sneezing, congestion, coughing, headache), stay home and take care of yourself. The sooner you boost your immune system and get rid of the bug that "bit" you, the sooner you can resume your regular schedule.

USE AN HERBAL BOOSTER: As a preventive measure, you can keep your immune system in good shape by supplementing echinacea (25 drops of tincture once or twice daily) and stinging nettle (a cup of dried leaf infusion daily, and add seaweeds, such as kelp or wakame, to soups, stews, and casseroles.

GET AN X RAY AND DIAGNOSIS: If you have walking pneumonia, you may not think that much is the matter with you and ignore your symptoms. That can be dangerous. For this reason, if you have a persistent cough and chest pain, you should have an X ray taken of your lungs so that your doctor can make a diagnosis and prescribe the appropriate treatment.

STAY PUT: There is nothing much to do for viral pneumonia but go to bed, keep warm, and drink fluids. Bacterial pneumonia also requires bed rest in addition to antibiotics.

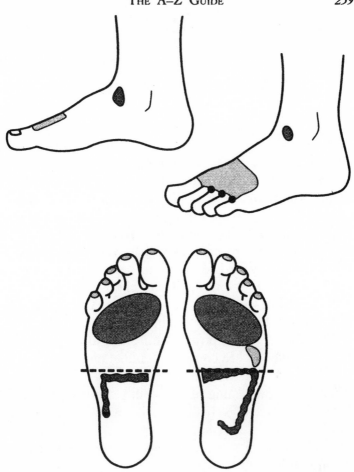

Pneumonia can be very serious—even life-threatening—in the elderly and the very young and requires medical care. Antibiotic treatment is almost always necessary with bacterial pneumonia and may also be advised with viral pneumonia in order to stave off secondary infections. Reflexology and the alternative treatments listed above will help increase energy in your system as you heal.

Postpartum Recovery

It's been weeks since the baby was born, but you still have trouble getting out of bed in the morning. Your breasts ache, and your episiotomy or tear makes going to the bathroom difficult. You're weepy and depressed about everything, from a bill in the mail to a wet diaper.

Your body has been through a great deal for the past nine months, and its culmination in either a natural or Caesarean delivery can leave you sore and upset. It takes time for your breasts to accommodate to nursing (or to the milk drying up if you choose not to nurse), and the entire vaginal/anal area or your Caesarean incision may be too sore to touch.

It's normal to get postpartum blues after a delivery. Hormonal levels are completely unbalanced and will be for quite a while, and the stress of daily life and your sense of overwhelming responsibility can lead to a lot of problematic feelings. It's harder if you have no real support system: a participative partner, a mother or mother-in-law or sister, or neighbors who can help out when you need it.

SYMPTOMS: Sore, aching breasts with leaking milk; pain or itching in the vaginal/anal area or around the incision site. In addition, a persistent blue feeling, great fatigue, loss of interest in your child. You may be agitated, confused, hypersensitive with feelings of paranoia, having obsessional or repetitive thoughts, loss of appetite, and difficulty sleeping.

AREAS TO TREAT/TYPES OF MANIPULATION

Work both feet completely first. Then find the locations of reflexes that correspond to these organs, and work in the following order (see Chapter 3 for guidance):

1. Uterus: Apply gradual circular pressure with thumb tip and pad.
2. Ovaries: Apply gradual circular pressure with thumb tip and pad.
3. Fallopian Tubes: Glide thumb tip back and forth across area.
4. Hips: Work thumb edge all around lower edge of outer anklebone.
5. Kidneys: Apply direct pressure with thumb tip.
6. Adrenals: Apply direct pressure with thumb tip.

PREVENTIVE MEASURES AND COMPLEMENTARY TREATMENTS

Reflexology works well in conjunction with other alternative therapies and commonsense measures. For example:

GET HELP: It's vital to have some backup with a new baby: a relative or friend to do some shopping, take care of your other children, and give you a break so you can get out alone for a walk. If you have no close relations or friends nearby, perhaps you can arrange a "swap" with a neighbor who also has young children.

GET OUT AND EXERCISE: Some daily routine, such as walking, biking, and swimming, will get you back in your prepregnant shape faster, will give you much-needed private time away from your baby, and will trigger the production of the beta-endorphins in your brain that will restore your sense of well-being.

HERBS TO SLOW BLEEDING: In order to slow postpartum lochia, or bloody discharge, take 15 to 30 drops of shep-

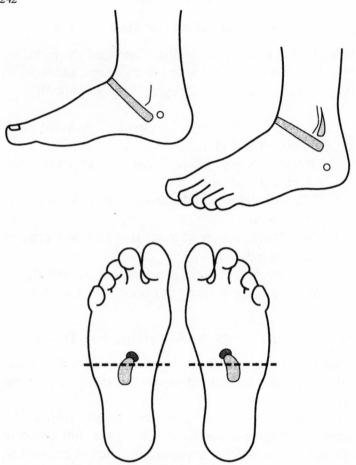

herd's purse, witch hazel, blue or black cohosh, or trillium four times daily.

HELP FOR YOUR BREASTS: If they're engorged, frequent nursing and expressing will give relief. You can also stand under a warm shower and let the milk leak out. If your nipples are cracked, make sure you don't use soap on them; it will dry them out further. Instead wash with plain water, pat dry, then apply calendula cream.

HELP FOR YOUR VAGINAL DISCOMFORT: To take down swelling of the vaginal area after a tear or episiotomy, sit several times daily in a sitz bath that contains a handful of comfrey leaves. You can also visualize the area drawing together with imaginary knitting needles made of soft rubber.

You should remain in telephone contact with your obstetrician after the birth and be scheduled for a six-week checkup postpartum. However, if reflexology and the alternative therapies listed above have not alleviated your postpartum blues, vaginal healing, and breast-feeding difficulties, or if you are bleeding copiously, see your physician at once.

PROSTATE PROBLEMS

You never used to get up in the middle of the night; now you're awakened three times to urinate. It's difficult to get the stream started, and when it finally does, there's some blood in it.

The prostate is a doughnut-shaped gland that sits at the base of the penis and encircles the urethra. Its function is to secrete an alkaline substance that makes up part of the seminal fluid, which protects the sperm and gives it mobility. The gland is about the size of a walnut from birth through the start of midlife, although it enlarges in later life. It is also subject to infections, which may spread from the bladder. Abnormal growth of cells in this gland can develop into cancer.

Prostatism is an enlargement of the prostate gland, which constricts the urethra, making urination difficult. It is hard to start a flow, and even after it's begun, there may be only a few drops, leaving the bladder full. More frequent urination (day and night) is usually necessary. This condition generally occurs in men over fifty and often requires surgery to remove part of the gland and alleviate the pressure on the urethra.

Prostatitis is an irritating infection of the gland that may result when the bladder remains full because the enlarged prostate does not permit passage of a complete flow of urine. It may become very uncomfortable to urinate, and other symptoms of infection (fever, chills, etc.) may result.

The second most common cancer in men after lung cancer is prostate cancer, which occurs mainly over the age of fifty-five. Heredity may play some part in the development of this cancer, but the actual cause is not known. Generally the cancer develops slowly, without symptoms, and is picked up only on a self-exam or physician's exam when a lump is detected in the prostate. A digital rectal exam (DRE) and new diagnostic blood test (PSA, or prostate-specific antigen) should be performed yearly from the age of fifty on. The blood test is not completely accurate, however, and there are many false positives and negatives.

If your cancer is detected in the early stages, there is a good survival rate after surgery to remove the entire gland and surrounding lymph nodes or radiation, or both. If the cancer has spread, hormones may help slow the tumor's growth. Cryosurgery (freezing the gland) is a new treatment offered, but it is still in experimental stages.

SYMPTOMS: *Prostatism:* You may have difficulty beginning the stream of urine, decreased force, and only a few droplets at the end; occasionally there may be blood in the urine.

Prostatitis: You may feel a fullness in the lower back and pelvic region, a burning sensation while urinating, fever, and chills.

Prostate cancer: Usually there are no symptoms. In advanced cases, when the cancer has spread to the bone, there may be pain in the bones.

AREAS TO TREAT/TYPES OF MANIPULATION

Work both feet completely first. Then find the locations of reflexes that correspond to these organs, and work in the following order (see Chapter 3 for guidance):

1. Testes: Apply direct circular pressure with thumb tip and pad.
2. Prostate: Apply gradual circular pressure with thumb tip and pad.
3. Lymph Glands: Work thumb pad and tip gently back and forth across area.
4. Groin: Apply firm thumb pressure throughout bottom of heel.
4. Lower Back (Lumbar Spine): Glide thumb tip down the inside of the foot from the base of the ball to the top of the heel.
5. Bladder: Apply circular pressure with thumb pad.

PREVENTIVE MEASURES AND COMPLEMENTARY TREATMENTS

Reflexology works well in conjunction with other alternative therapies and commonsense measures. For example:

GET A CHECKUP: Every man over fifty should have a yearly regular medical checkup, including a digital rectal exam and an examination of the penis, testes, and prostate.

URINATE WHEN YOU HAVE TO: In order to avoid bladder infections, which may lead to prostate infections, it's vital to urinate when you feel the urge. If you are having

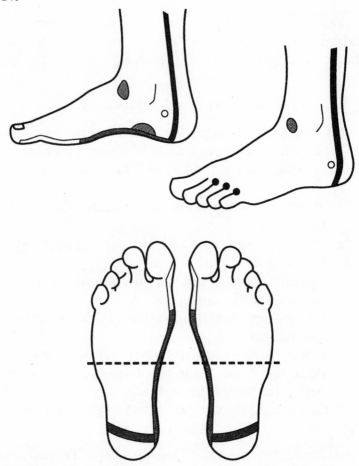

trouble with the flow, you can turn on some water, or visualize water running.

EAT LOW FAT: Since dietary fat may stimulate excessive hormonal production, a low-fat diet is currently believed to be beneficial in the prevention of several cancers, particularly breast, colon, and prostate cancer.

If you are having difficulty urinating or see blood in your urine, you should see your physician. Reflexology and commonsense treatments may assist in clearing blockages in the genital area.

PSORIASIS

It's as if you were a fish losing scales. You are always sure that the rash that's dried up and flaked off is over with, and then the scales re-form. And they're all over your body, so there's no escape.

This hereditary skin condition seems to be caused by a lack of ability of the skin to handle injury and inflammation as well as a deregulation of cells that provide immune protection. Research that's been done on people with psoriasis shows that epidermal cell division and keratinizing (scaling off) occurs much more quickly than with normal cells.

Some individuals with psoriasis develop a related condition similar to rheumatoid arthritis. It can be mild and cause occasional swelling of fingers and toes, or it can be crippling, affecting the spine, hips, and shoulders.

SYMPTOMS: The outbreaks generally start with a small red papule covered with an almost transparent scale. This then escalates to a red patch several inches around covered with silvery white scales that flake off and re-form. They may appear on the elbows, the knees, the scalp (causing bald patches), the nails, even the genitals.

AREAS TO TREAT/TYPES OF MANIPULATION

Work both feet completely first. Then find the locations of reflexes that correspond to these organs, and work in the following order (see Chapter 3 for guidance):

1. Kidneys: Apply direct pressure with thumb tip.
2. Thyroid: Work "necks" of toes with thumb tip.

3. Adrenals: Apply direct pressure with thumb tip.
4. Pituitary: Apply direct pressure with thumb tip.

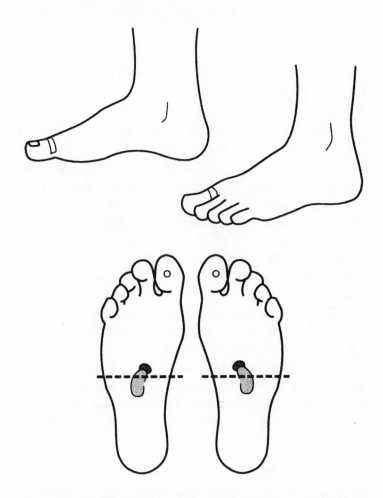

PREVENTIVE MEASURES AND COMPLEMENTARY TREATMENTS

Reflexology works well in conjunction with other alternative therapies and commonsense measures. For example:

BE GENTLE: Since anything from a bump on the elbow

to clothing that rubs a portion of skin can trigger an outbreak, it's important to be careful with yourself. Don't wear a tight waistband that might cause friction, and avoid activities like rock climbing or contact sports that might injure your skin.

TRY A LOTION: Various corticosteroid creams and ointments are often prescribed, although they can cause side effects and must be carefully monitored by a physician. Another type of medication called anthralin, processed from crude coal tar, is an effective form of treatment, although it temporarily discolors and can sometimes irritate the skin.

SEEK THE LIGHT: Ultraviolet A light therapy combined with an oral medication, psoralen, that sensitizes the skin to the UV rays, is a widely used and very effective treatment. PUVA (the acronym that mixes the name of the drug and the UV rays) can cause skin burning and must be carefully administered. It is still controversial whether the therapy may put users at higher risk for skin cancer in later life.

If you have severe psoriasis, it is advisable to consult a physician who will prescribe corticosteroids, methotrexate (a drug in cancer chemotherapy), or etretinate, a very powerful vitamin A derivative that is used when all other treatments fail. Reflexology and the alternative treatments listed above may alleviate symptoms so that you and your doctor will be able to reduce the amount of your medication or therapy.

Sciatica (see also Back Problems, p. 70)

The pain runs from your buttock down the back of your leg to your heel. Sometimes it's a mild discomfort; at other times you're in exquisite pain.

Sciatica is an inflammation of the sciatic nerve, which runs down from the lower back across the buttock to the outside of the thigh, then down the leg to the foot. Anything that causes pressure on this nerve, from lumbar disk damage to lifting weights or twisting the spine by sitting with legs crossed all the time, may cause a range of discomfort, from slight annoyance to excruciating agony. It all depends how far the injured disk has been displaced and how directly it presses on the nerve. You may feel perfectly fine one minute, then sneeze, causing the disk to press suddenly on the nerve, sending you up the wall. If the disk ruptures, an inflammation of the nerve can set in that causes constant and considerable pain, as well as numbness of the entire area.

SYMPTOMS: Pain, which may be slight or severe, down the back of the leg from the buttock to the heel. Additional twinges may occur on coughing or sneezing. Numbness or pins and needles tingling down the leg.

Areas to Treat/Types of Manipulation

Work both feet completely first. Then find the locations of reflexes that correspond to these organs, and work in the following order (see Chapter 3 for guidance):

1. Hip/Sciatic Nerve: Work thumb edge all around lower edge of outer anklebone.
2. Groin: Apply firm thumb pressure throughout bottom of heel.
3. Lymph Glands: Work thumb tip and pad gently back and forth across area of reflex.
4. Lower Back (Lumbar Spine): Glide thumb down inside of foot from base of the ball to the top of the heel.
5. Tailbone (Coccyx): Apply gentle circular pressure with thumb tip.
6. Knees: Work the end of the thumb all around the fifth metatarsal bone on the outside of each foot.

PREVENTIVE MEASURES AND COMPLEMENTARY TREATMENTS

Reflexology works well in conjunction with other alternative therapies and commonsense measures. For example:

TAKE A REST: It's best to stay off your feet and not try too much activity, which you probably won't want to do anyway. Lie flat on a firm mattress as much as possible; stay off soft couches, which will be difficult to get into and out of and harmful to your back while you're there.

BRING YOUR KNEES TO YOUR CHEST: Lie on the floor, and hug your knees into your chest only as far as is comfortable. Now, using resistance, pull the knees apart with your hands; then push them back together, as though there were weights attached to your legs that made them difficult to move. Using tension and pressure during this movement pushes the sciatic nerve into place.

GET IN THE WATER: Hydrotherapy, in which a stream of water is directed at the nerve, is often employed by physical therapists to treat sciatica.

DO TAI CHI CHUAN: The gentle, slow movements of this ancient Chinese meditative practice allow the spine to

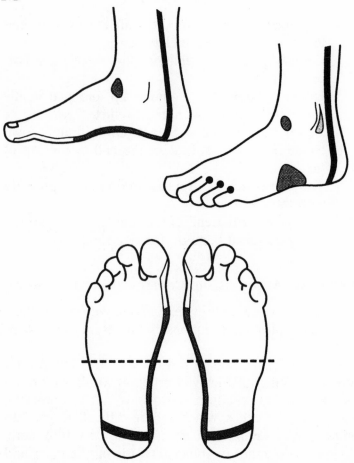

realign itself for optimum health. The working structural concept in tai chi chuan, of being "suspended from above," as though you were a marionette on strings, helps keep all the vertebrae, and the nerves within the spinal column, in line. Daily practice will help develop the core muscles (the four muscle groups that form the waist) and takes the pressure off the lumbar spine.

Reflexology and the alternative treatments listed above will alleviate pain and help you strengthen your back. However, if your sciatic pain persists, or if you have constant numbness in your leg and foot, you may have a ruptured disk and should consult a physician.

Sexual Dysfunction (see also Impotence, p. 197)

You are attracted, but you're scared. You think about sex constantly, yet you're filled with apprehension about losing control. Or perhaps you had a traumatic experience, such as rape or abuse, and you don't want anything to do with sex.

Problems relating to sexuality are rampant in our society. Although sex is all around us—in movies, MTV videos, in our music and advertising—most of us grow up with a variety of sexual limitations. We may have felt enormous confusion about whether we felt allegiance to our own sex or the other; we may have been admonished in childhood for touching ourselves or another child; we may have learned too young what sex was all about because of the horror of childhood incest or abuse. Family, peers, school, and religious upbringing all figure in our various adaptations to the sexual nature we're all born with.

If you're like most people, your sexual feelings are intimately related to your ability to love and give to another. Yet it's just as possible to feel affection and fondness without having sex enter into the picture as it is to feel physical passion for someone you don't really like very much. The differences in your fantasies and your willingness to confront what Eros actually means to you can set off feelings of loneliness and depression. You can't reach out because you're afraid you want too much.

These frustrating and difficult concerns may rear their head in the bedroom. If you don't communicate what you want or what you're afraid of, and you're a woman, you may not have an orgasm, or penetrative sex may be excruciatingly painful for you. If you're a man, you may not be able to achieve or maintain an erection. If these problems occur too often, you may turn off sex completely and find that you are numb to any previously exciting stimulus.

The feelings of shame and humiliation we may have about our sexual needs can easily color other aspects of our relationships. For this reason, it's vital to try to balance energies that may be blocked or stunted in both mind and body.

SYMPTOMS: Impotence (erectile dysfunction), anorgasmia (inability to have an orgasm), dyspareunia (pain with intercourse), shame/humiliation about the body, compulsive sexual fantasies, sexual numbness.

AREAS TO TREAT/TYPES OF MANIPULATION

Work both feet completely first. Then find the locations of reflexes that correspond to these organs, and work in the following order (see Chapter 3 for guidance):

1. Solar Plexus: With thumb tip, apply gradual pressure in the middle of the reflex, and work out to the edges.
2. Endocrine Glands (Adrenals, Thyroid/Parathyroid, Pituitary)
   Adrenals: Apply direct pressure with thumb tip.
   Thyroid/Parathyroid: Work "necks" of toes with thumb tip.

Pituitary: Apply direct pressure with thumb tip.
3. Reproductive System: Apply gradual circular pressure with thumb tip and pad to ovaries and uterus (female) or prostate and testes (male).

PREVENTIVE MEASURES AND COMPLEMENTARY TREATMENTS

Reflexology works well in conjunction with other alternative therapies and commonsense measures. For example:

START TALKING: The more you let each other know what you're feeling and what you'd like to do and refrain from doing, the better your sexual functioning will be. Try having a conversation about your desires and fears outside the bedroom, to take the pressure off. A long car ride together or a picnic by a quiet lake may let you open up and clear the air.

TRY A CHINESE HERB: The patent formula gou ji dze jiou, Chinese wolfberry wine, available in Chinese tea and herb shops (in most Chinatowns) or by mail order, is an herbal tonic that boosts sexual functioning for both men and women. A stimulant to the liver and kidney, this tonic stimulates the production of hormones, blood, and enzymes throughout the body. Take one or two doses of 1.5 oz. daily on an empty stomach.

FIND OUT WHAT GIVES YOU PLEASURE: When you're concerned about performing for a partner, you don't give yourself ample time to relax and enjoy sex. Take an evening alone to sit in a warm tub with a glass of wine or cup of tea, listening to music. Touch your body and relish the sensations you get. Masturbation can serve as a teaching tool, letting you know just what excites you and what turns you off. Using it judiciously can help in your partnered sexual relationship as well.

DO YOUR EXERCISES: Kegel exercises can help both men and women recapture the feeling of arousal. To do a

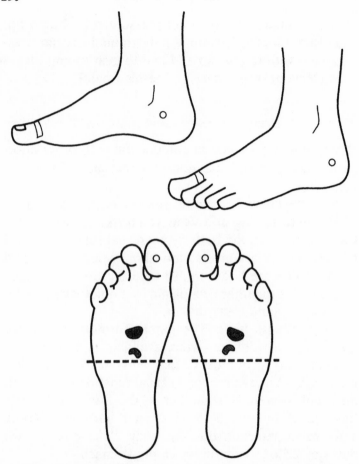

Kegel, pretend that you are sitting on the toilet if you're a woman, standing if you're a man, letting out the flow of urine. Then, using the muscles around the urethra and vagina or penis, stop the flow. (Men will see their testicles pull up toward the body as they clench these muscles.) Practice three sets of ten, three times daily, for increased control and stimulation.

GET OFF MEDICATION: Various drugs, from antihistamines to mood-altering medications, can dampen your ardor. The worst offenders are high blood pressure medications; ask your doctor if you can change brands or reduce the dosage. Many antidepressants and drugs similar to Prozac also reduce sex drive, so you may want to consider weaning yourself off these slowly. The sexual act itself produces lots of serotonin, the neurotransmitter that fills us with a sense of delight and well-being.

If reflexology and the alternative treatments listed above have not improved your sexual functioning after several months, consult your physician, who may recommend a sex therapist, urologist, or psychologist, depending on your particular problem.

SHOULDER PAIN (SEE ALSO ARTHRITIS, P. 62; BURSITIS, P. 86)

It feels as if you've got the world on your shoulders because your whole body seems focused on the pain in this joint. The shoulder joint, a ball and socket, allows movement in many directions. Because of the freedom possible in the range of lifting, lowering, moving back and forth, and turning in a complete circle, the joint relies heavily on the ligaments that support it. However, these ligaments and the surrounding muscles are generally weak relative to the capacity of the joint. This means that the shoulder can be easily damaged or injured.

If you pull the joint out of its normal position, you get a dislocation, which is the most common shoulder injury.

Damage to a joint creates wear and tear over the

years; this may result in arthritis. And inflammation from sudden pressure or continual use of the shoulder joint may damage the shock-absorbing sacs of fluid that protect the joint (the bursas), resulting in bursitis.

Because the shoulder is so versatile in its movement, the many muscles that interact to create shoulder motion are sometimes in jeopardy. The four muscles of the rotator cuff, which attach to the front, rear, top, and head of the humerus (the long bone from the elbow to the shoulder), are easily torn during any kind of strenuous activity. If you throw all your energy into playing baseball, basketball, football, or any racquet sport, it shouldn't be surprising if you tear a rotator cuff.

You may also have a frozen shoulder, either from a badly healed rotator cuff, or from any type of repetitive motion using this joint, such as painting a ceiling, too much gardening or tennis, or pulling heavy grocery bags out of carts. The problem arises when you start to favor the injured arm. The capsule that covers the shoulder joint has to be moved around in order to function properly, and when it stays in one position too long, portions of this sleeve can stick together, forming adhesions— like poorly healed scar tissue. At this point, when you try to move it, it feels stuck, so you don't exercise it, and it becomes immobilized.

SYMPTOMS: *Dislocation or Torn Rotator Cuff:* Sharp pain in the shoulder, restriction or loss of movement in one or all directions.

Arthritis: pain, swelling, redness, tenderness of joint, restriction of movement, particularly in damp weather.

Bursitis: pain, swelling, fluid around joint, restriction of movement.

Frozen Shoulder: complete restriction of movement, pain with movement.

AREAS TO TREAT/TYPES OF MANIPULATION

Work both feet completely first. Then find the locations of reflexes that correspond to these organs, and work in the following order (see Chapter 3 for guidance):

1. Shoulder: Apply firm circular pressure to reflex with thumb tip.
2. Neck: Using thumb and index finger, manipulate "necks" of toes thoroughly.
3. Mid-back (Thoracic Spine): Glide thumb down the inside of the foot from the base of the big toe to the bottom of the ball.
4. Hips: Work edge of thumb all around lower edge of outer anklebone.

PREVENTIVE MEASURES AND COMPLEMENTARY TREATMENTS

Reflexology works well in conjunction with other alternative therapies and commonsense measures. For example:

TRY R.I.C.E.: The combination of rest, ice, compression, and elevation is best for inflamed joints and ligaments. Wrap an Ace bandage around your arm and shoulder, place an ice bag around the affected area, and prop pillows under you.

USE HEAT IF YOUR SHOULDER FREEZES: Apply a warm heating pad to allow the muscles to relax and extend. If your condition is very serious, you may have to consult an orthopedist, who will heat the area with ultrasound aimed into the shoulder joint.

KEEP IT IN A SLING: Especially if the injured shoulder is on your primary side, you will need to keep it immobilized at times when you aren't training it therapeutically. While at your desk, walking down the street, or sitting listening to music or watching television, put a sling

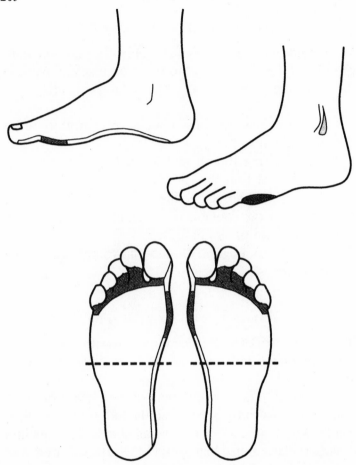

around your neck and keep the arm inside it. Feeling this physical restriction will keep you from accidentally injuring it again.

EXPERIMENT WITH MOVEMENT: Gently, carrying your injured arm with your good arm as though it were on a tray, try out your range of movement. Lift it a few inches, bring it forward, to the side, backward, and to the other side. One movement therapy that is particularly beneficial as you recuperate is Feldenkrais, in which you are guided by a practitioner to use one part of your body as though you had never used it before. You can find Feldenkrais instruction in most urban areas through holistic centers or body/mind classes at your local Y.

If your shoulder is terribly painful and your movement is extremely restricted, consult your physician. A torn rotator cuff may require surgery, after which time reflexology and commonsense measures will help you to heal more quickly and efficiently.

Sinusitis

Oh, the pressure in your head. It's as if an elephant had somehow found its way inside the bones of your face and skull.

Sinusitis is an infection of one or more of the mucous membranes lining the sinuses, the air-filled cavities inside the facial bone structure, connected to the nose. There are four groups of sinuses: the ethmoidal and frontal sinuses above each brow, and the maxillary and sphenoidal sinuses on either side of the nose below the cheekbones.

If your sinuses are functioning normally, mucus drains through them into the nasal passages. When you have a cold or the flu, these passages become congested, and the mucus stays blocked in the sinus cavities where bacteria breed, causing infection. They can also become inflamed from swimming or diving, allergies, an abscessed tooth, or an injury to the face.

My client Janet's sinuses were so congested she had headaches most of the time. Before I met her, she'd been living on over-the-counter decongestants, which dried out all her mucous membranes (not just her sinuses) and gave only temporary relief. So we started working together, concentrating on her sinuses, her entire head and neck, her eyes and ears, her kidneys and adrenals. During the first treatment her breathing became noticeably easier, and continued self-treatment on her sinus reflex points kept her problem under control without medication.

SYMPTOMS: Pain and tenderness of the face and forehead, the eyes, top of the nose, and top teeth. You may also have headaches, chills, fever, clogged nasal passages, and some yellow greenish mucus discharged from the nose. The discomfort is often negligible on arising but gets worse throughout the day.

AREAS TO TREAT/TYPES OF MANIPULATION

Work both feet completely first. Then find the locations of reflexes that correspond to these organs, and work in the following order (see Chapter 3 for guidance):

1. Sinus: Using thumb tip, first work the tips of the toes, using a circular motion; then work all around the whole toe.
2. Neck: Using thumb and index finger, manipulate "necks" of toes thoroughly.
3. Ileocecal Valve: Apply direct pressure with thumb tip.
4. Adrenals: Apply direct pressure with thumb tip.
5. Pituitary: Apply direct pressure with thumb tip.

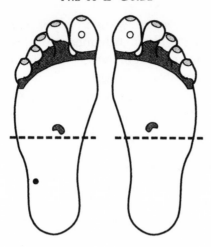

PREVENTIVE MEASURES AND COMPLEMENTARY TREATMENTS

Reflexology works well in conjunction with other alternative therapies and commonsense measures. For example:

DRAIN YOUR MUCUS: You can stand in a hot shower or stick your head over a pot of chamomile tea with a towel draped over your head. You can also get good drainage with a salt-water solution. Mix 1 teaspoon salt with 2 cups of warm water; put the mixture into a dropper and squeeze it into each nostril; allow the water to run out in the sink. Repeat several times in both nostrils.

COOK WITH CAYENNE: Cayenne pepper will get your nasal secretions running and open sinus passages. The pepper contains capsaicin, which stimulates nerve fibers and acts as a natural decongestant.

DRINK LOTS OF FLUIDS: Flushing the system with liquids thins the mucus so that it can move more easily. Certain herbs—fenugreek, anise, fennel, and sage—also stimulate mucus drainage.

DON'T USE NASAL SPRAYS: The sprays shrink the mucous membranes, but since the infection is still present, they tend to swell even more than before you sprayed. This vicious cycle ends only when you stop using the sprays.

If reflexology and other natural treatments haven't helped the pain and pressure, consult a physician, who may prescribe antibiotics or may drain your sinuses manually. Certain chronic blockages may require surgery, but reflexology will help in speeding the healing process.

SKIN DISORDERS (SEE ALSO ACNE, P. 42; ECZEMA, P. 122; PSORIASIS, P. 247)

You can't look in the mirror, and you can't face the day. When there's an eruption anywhere on your body, be it a pimple, wart, poison ivy, or sunburn, it's hard to feel at your best.

The skin is the largest organ of the body, covering about two square yards (in an average-size man) and weighing over ten pounds. There are two layers: the epidermis on top and the dermis (with its network of blood vessels, sebaceous and sweat glands, and hair shafts and follicles) beneath. Under these is a layer of subcutaneous fat. The epidermis, made of twenty layers of cells, is constantly turning over, because of cell division, so that you gain a new upper skin about every month (this process is faster in children and slower in the elderly).

As the skin ages, the dermis, which is made up of connective tissue, becomes less elastic and more fragile. It is also more prone to discoloration from greater production of melanin, a darkly pigmented material formed by a particular type of skin cell called a melanocyte.

This organ may suffer disruptions in the functioning of any number of processes: dilation of blood vessels that inflame the skin and then cause it to "weep" (dermatitis), which may be caused by anything from a burn to the ill effects of poison ivy or poison oak sap, the separation of the dermis and epidermis (as in a tennis blister caused by traumatizing the area over and over), or the proliferation of abnormal cells (melanoma).

SYMPTOMS: Various skin disorders will create rashes, blisters or abrasions, or general disruptions of epidermal tissue that may be red, purple, yellow-green, or blue-black. They may itch or be extremely painful; they may be hot to the touch. Some may stay localized in one spot; others will spread if not carefully treated and monitored.

Dermatitis: An inflammation of the epidermis. First, the small blood vessels become engorged and dilated, allowing fluid to leave the vessels and accumulate in the tissue. As the tissue swells, it forms blisters, which may break open and weep. Some dermatitis does not create

blisters but instead causes redness, scaling, and thickening of the skin. Dermatitis can be caused by chemical
irritants (detergents, ammonia, turpentine, etc.), dry
skin, poor circulation (thrombophlebitis or varicose
veins that may cause skin ulcers), eczema, which thickens and discolors the skin or causes a red blistering rash,
or allergic contact dermatitis, which occurs when the
skin comes into contact with an allergen such as poison
ivy, oak, or sumac.

Allergic Contact Dermatitis: A red blistering rash that
occurs only where the skin has touched the sap of the
poison ivy, oak, or sumac plant. The rash usually appears twenty-four to forty-eight hours after contact and
develops into large, fluid-filled blisters, which weep
and eventually crust over. There may also be swelling
and redness around the eyes if you happened to touch
that area after contact with the plant. Although one blister cannot spread to another area, you may reinfect
yourself if you don't get the sap out from under your
fingernails after your first contact. The excruciating itching reaction may last two to three weeks, and it may
take months to have completely clear new skin after a
bad case.

Other Skin Allergies: Metal (particularly nickel), rubber, hair dye, and cosmetics all may cause allergic reactions, as can drugs and exposure to the sun. These range
from itching and redness to swelling and blistering.
Some food and drug allergies create hives, which are
itchy, red, or skin-colored raised areas that resemble
insect bites.

Most of these allergies are unpleasant but disappear
by themselves as soon as contact with the allergen is
removed.

Bacterial Skin Infections: These include folliculitis and
boils.

Folliculitis is caused by *Staphylococcus* bacteria in the opening of a hair follicle, which can create a small pus pimple with a red area around it. This often happens during shaving.

Another staph infection, a boil, is a painful deep red nodule, an inflammation of the hair follicle and the surrounding skin. The back of the neck and under the armpit are common places for boils to develop. Generally a boil comes to a head and discharges pus, after which it will shrink and become absorbed back into the skin. Persistent boils require antibiotic therapy.

Viral Skin Infections: These are herpes simplex, warts, and shingles.

The herpes simplex virus can remain dormant in the body for years until triggered by heat (sun exposure or fever), illness, emotional stress, the menstrual cycle, or certain medications. When the virus is active, the symptoms are a rash of several small, swollen red blisters (a cold sore or fever blister are two manifestations of herpes). When active, herpes is contagious. However, as the blisters crust over and heal, the virus cannot be transmitted to another.

Warts, caused by an infectious virus, are irregular nodules with many small blood vessels that look like black dots. They bleed easily and can be spread around the body and from person to person. They often regrow even after treatment (by freezing, surgery, or acid treatments) because a wart may vanish but the virus is much harder to eradicate.

Shingles—red, swollen clusters of blisters on the torso or face as well as an inflammation of the nerves that produces a pins-and-needles sensation—is a painful condition caused by the same virus that causes chicken pox. Experts think that after a childhood bout of pox the virus remains in the body attached to a spinal nerve root, where it can break out years later.

Fungal Skin Infections: These include ringworm and yeast infections.

The fungus that causes ringworm creates a path of red, scaly skin, distinct from the healthy skin because of its elevated, rounded border. It can be seen on particular areas of the body: in the groin area as jock itch and between the toes as athlete's foot. It may also be present in the scalp and nails.

The fungus known as *Candida albicans* can create the common cheesy vaginal discharge as well as sores at the corners of the mouth and inside the cheeks, swelling and redness around the nails, and moist red rashes on the body. Certain groups of individuals are more susceptible to this virus than others—for example, diabetics, people with endocrine disorders, women on birth control pills or tetracycline, and babies (who wear diapers).

Sunburn: The sun emits two types of radiation: the short, high-energy rays that produce sunburn (ultraviolet B, or UVB) and the long, low-energy waves that tan and also produce sun-allergic reactions (ultraviolet A, or UVA). In order to prevent skin damage, it's important either to reduce the time spent in the presence of both types of rays or to guard against their effect with repeated applications of sunblock.

Sunburn initially shows up as redness, followed by pain, heat, sensitivity to touch, and sometimes swelling of tissues. After twenty-four to forty-eight hours, the skin begins to peel, and after that, the melanin in the epidermal cells is oxidized from brown to darker brown, and the melanocytes produce increased amounts of melanin, which causes a tan (some types of skin never tan, but only stay red). A suntan is the mechanism the body uses to protect itself from further overexposure to radiation—that is, it's not a healthy state for the skin to be in.

Skin Cancer/Melanomas: Chronic exposure to the sun is the major cause of skin cancer, although it can also be caused by environmental damage from radiation exposure. Basal cell cancer is the most common and is sometimes but not always seen as a pinkish, smooth-surfaced, solid group of cells that bleeds easily. This type of cancer may grow deep into the skin but will not spread to the bloodstream or lymph system and can be treated with surgery, chemotherapy, and radiation. Squamous cell carcinomas may begin as precancerous red, scaly lesions on sun-damaged, burned, or radiation-poisoned skin and may grow into crusted, heaped-up nodules. These cancers are generally treated surgically. Malignant melanoma, a pigment cell cancer, is the most dangerous of all types of skin cancer and may result in death if not detected early and treated aggressively. These melanomas resemble moles but with several differences: They are asymmetrical, they have scalloped borders, and they are multicolored. You should see your physician at once if a preexisting mole has begun to change in shape, elevation, sensation, or consistency, or if the skin surrounding it has become red or swollen.

AREAS TO TREAT/TYPE OF MANIPULATION

Work both feet completely first. Then find the locations of reflexes that correspond to these organs, and work in the following order (see Chapter 3 for guidance):

1. Kidneys: Apply direct pressure with thumb tip.
2. Thyroid: Work "necks" of toes with thumb tip.
3. Reproductive System: Apply gradual circular pressure with thumb tip and pad to ovaries and uterus (female) or prostate and testes (male).

4. Adrenals: Apply direct pressure with thumb tip.
5. Pituitary: Apply direct pressure with thumb tip.

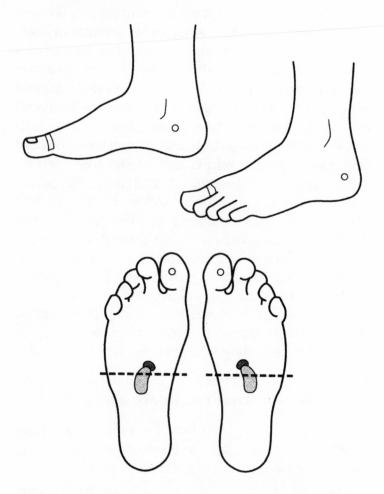

PREVENTIVE MEASURES AND COMPLEMENTARY TREATMENTS

Reflexology works well in conjunction with other alternative therapies and commonsense measures. For example:

KNOW YOUR ALLERGIES: If you periodically break out in

hives, that's a good sign that you should try to avoid certain foods or drugs. Try cutting out chocolate, nuts, eggs, pork, penicillin, and all chemical additives, like preservatives, dyes, and artificial flavorings.

PAY ATTENTION TO YOUR SURROUNDINGS: If you're walking in the woods (or just mowing your backyard), know that three shiny leaves mean poison ivy, which means TROUBLE. If you're on the beach, look down for jellyfish. If you're out on a picnic, be on the lookout for wasps and bees.

TAKE A COOL BATH WITH BAKING SODA: This combination can alleviate the itching and swelling prevalent in dermatitis.

USE CUCUMBERS: If you have a relatively small, localized itching or painful area, one of the best and most cooling treatments is a poultice of cucumber slices.

CREATE A SKIN HYGIENE ROUTINE: Be sure you pay attention to your skin daily, washing it with warm water and soap, getting rid of dead skin with a loofah scrub, and eating plenty of fresh vegetables and fruits to provide it with the vitamins and minerals it needs. Also, be sure that you get sufficient sleep; a good eight hours a night will restore that glow.

STAY OUT OF THE SUN: To avoid a bad sunburn and particularly to prevent melanomas, the best advice is to avoid sunbathing completely. Remember that ultraviolet rays penetrate even on cloudy days. If you must be outside during the hottest time of day, cover up: Long sleeves and a hat are essential.

Reflexology and the other alternative treatments listed above will alleviate certain skin conditions and reduce the severity of others. However, infections and certain cancers must be treated medically. If you are at all confused about the type of lesion or eruption on your skin, consult a physician at once.

✳

Sore Throat

We all know that feeling: Your throat is on fire, and nothing will put out the flames. It hurts too much to swallow, and the scratchiness is unbearable.

A sore throat is usually the beginning of an upper respiratory infection, or cold. (It may also be the first symptom of flu or measles and a variety of childhood diseases.) It is an inflammation of the tissues lining the throat that can easily occur from either bacteria or viruses that may invade the system.

The back of the tongue, the tonsils, the pharynx, and the cavity beneath the nose are all subject to the passage of air, food, drink, and mucus coughed up from the lungs. This means that the risk of infection at this site is very high, and the same infection may spare the throat but attack the sinuses, giving you a runny or stuffy nose. A sore throat isn't necessarily caused by one particular germ but usually any one of a roving band, since this is an area that always has bacteria and other microorganisms present.

Sore throats may also stem from noninfectious causes, such as smoking, drinking a scalding liquid, or discharge from the sinuses that runs down the back of the throat.

SYMPTOMS: The sore throat itself is the symptom of a certain type of infection. The most common type of sore throat, pharyngitis, is a viral infection of the pharynx, the area of the throat farthest back in the mouth. It generally starts with a feeling of dryness and irritation. You may have pain when you swallow, and you may find it hard to clear the mucus as you do. The condition usually lasts several days to a week.

AREAS TO TREAT/TYPES OF MANIPULATION

Work both feet completely first. Then find the locations of reflexes that correspond to these organs, and work in the following order (see Chapter 3 for guidance):

1. Throat: Apply gradual, direct pressure on the throat reflex. (CAUTION: This may be painful.)
2. Neck: Using thumb and index finger, manipulate "necks" of toes thoroughly.
3. Adrenals: Apply direct pressure with thumb tip.
4. Lymph Glands: Work thumb tip and pad gently back and forth across area.

PREVENTIVE MEASURES AND COMPLEMENTARY TREATMENTS

Reflexology works well in conjunction with other alternative therapies and commonsense measures. For example:

GARGLE WITH SALT: Put a teaspoon of salt into an 8-ounce glass of warm water, and gargle three to four times daily.

DRINK HOT FLUIDS: Take in as much herbal tea, chicken soup, and plain hot water with lemon as you can to soothe the area.

SUCK ON LOZENGES: Since you want to keep the throat as moist as possible, it's a good idea to suck on cough drops and throat lozenges.

DON'T TALK TOO MUCH: Talking brings in air, which, again, dries the throat and mucous membranes. So keep your mouth shut when your throat hurts!

If you have a persistent high fever (over 102) for more than four days, or if your throat has a yellow or

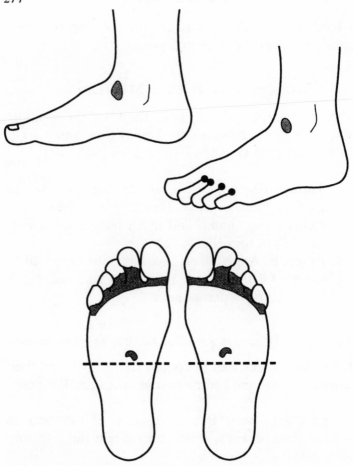

grayish coating, or you have great difficulty in swallowing, see a physician, who may wish to test for strep, ear infection, or tonsillitis.

STRAINS AND SPRAINS

You came off that last step a little funny, and now you're limping around. Maybe some repetitive motion, like throwing a ball or typing for a whole day, has made you twist your wrist. It's probably not serious enough for a trip to the emergency room, but it sure hurts.

A sprain results from an injury to a joint that damages the ligaments around it. You know immediately that you've done something wrong because it's excruciating, but you don't think you've broken anything. Sprains come in three grades: A Grade I injury involves minor damage to ligaments and the rupture of some small blood vessels. With a Grade II sprain, the ligament may be frayed, with a lot of blood vessel damage, and the joint may be unstable. A Grade III sprain involves the total rupture of a ligament and sometimes separation from the bone (many badly sprained ankles require casting).

Sprained ankles are the most common type of sprain, and some individuals are prone to them because of the way they walk. If you favor the outside of your foot, you tend to turn your ankle inward, and if you've already sprained your ankle, you may have loosened the outer ligaments, possibly making you prone to a second sprain.

A strain results from an injury between the muscle and the tendon (a few involve the tearing of tendon from the bone). With Grade I strains the muscle fiber is simply stretched out, and in a few days the discomfort dissipates. In a Grade II strain, many muscle fibers are torn, resulting in bleeding into the muscle tissue; muscle spasms are common. With Grade III the muscle ruptures; this type of injury requires complete immobilization for several months.

SYMPTOMS: *Sprain:* There is immediate pain, then bruising, tenderness, and swelling. A higher-grade sprain will make the symptoms more intense.

Strain: A slight strain will cause a few days of discomfort; a more serious one may result in muscle spasm reaction.

AREAS TO TREAT/TYPES OF MANIPULATION

Work both feet completely first. Then find the locations of reflexes that correspond to these organs, and work in the following order (see Chapter 3 for guidance):

1. Adrenals: Apply direct pressure with thumb tip.
2. Affected Body Part—that is, Ankle, Wrist, Knee, etc.: Do technique required on BOTH feet—that is, work same and opposite sides. Locate the area you need to treat on general chart of the foot, pp. 30–31.

PREVENTIVE MEASURES AND COMPLEMENTARY TREATMENTS

Reflexology works well in conjunction with other alternative therapies and commonsense measures. For example:

GET OFF THE INJURED AREA: If you've sprained your ankle, don't put weight on it. Let someone else help you to a chair or drive you home. Then prop the ankle up on cushions, and put an ice bag on it for twenty minutes out of every hour. (If it still hurts after two days, see a doctor for an X ray.)

DO YOUR EXERCISES: Physical therapy is essential in recuperating from strains and sprains. For stronger ankles, sit in a straight-backed chair and strap a one-

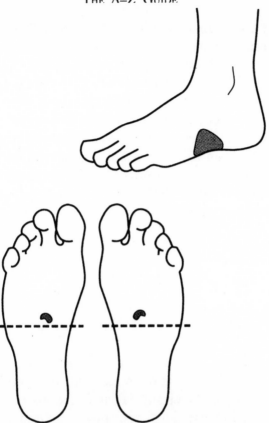

pound weight on top of your instep. Place a towel under your thigh as you flex and then relax your foot. Repeat twelve times. After a few weeks you can increase to a two-pound weight with eight repetitions. You can also do leg lifts, lying on your side on the floor, with the weight strapped on the outside of your injured foot below the anklebone.

You can do the same type of exercises for your wrist, but start out with a half-pound weight, and work your way up to one pound.

DON'T DO WHATEVER GAVE YOU THE PROBLEM: Running, jumping, climbing, etc. may lead to tripping, so if you're

healing a sore ankle, don't indulge. The activity leading
to a sprained wrist may not be as physical, but stay away
from repeating whatever it was that caused the injury.
When you're completely healed, you should perform
this activity in front of a physical therapist, who will be
able to point out the pitfalls of the movement and the
mistakes you've been making when you perform it.

If your sprain or strain is not improving after several
weeks of intensive reflexology and directed exercise, you
may have a fracture. See your physician for another set
of X rays and perhaps a cast.

STROKE

It may happen so quickly you don't even realize it. Or
you may be walking on the street with your mother and
suddenly see her reel and fall unconscious beside you.
All the basic senses split right down the middle: no vision in one eye, no feeling on one side. This event is
called a stroke.

A stroke takes place when sufficient blood flow cannot reach the brain and various areas in the brain are
deprived of oxygen. This causes a massive destruction of
brain cells, which can't be replaced. If the parts of the
brain affected are those that control speech, movement,
memory, or vision, the individual may lose those abilities partially or completely. The loss may be temporary
or permanent.

Although a stroke damages the brain, it is a cardiovascular event. Usually a stroke occurs because an ath-
erosclerotic plaque or clot forms in the brain or travels

there from elsewhere in the body. This event may accompany other cardiac problems; for example, the type of arrhythmia known as atrial fibrillation can set off the heart's pumping action so that it forms a clot that in turn travels to the brain. Open-heart surgery may also disrupt normal cardiac patterns and trigger a stroke.

There are several types of strokes: A cerebral hemorrhage occurs when a blood vessel in the brain ruptures. A particular type of hemorrhage is an aneurysm, when a weakened artery in the brain ruptures.

A cerebral embolism occurs when a blood clot travels from elsewhere in the body and blocks an artery that feeds the brain, while a cerebral thrombosis occurs when a clot (thrombosis) builds up on the wall of an artery leading from the heart to the brain and blocks blood flow to the brain.

Individuals who smoke, or who have diabetes, high blood pressure, or high cholesterol, have a higher risk of stroke than the general population.

SYMPTOMS: Some or all of the following may occur: You may feel dizzy and fall down; you may lose consciousness; you may suddenly lose vision in one eye; you may not be able to speak (aphasia) or understand others' speech; you may feel weak and numb down one side of your body or face; you may be paralyzed (hemiplegia).

There are also some individuals who get a warning attack, or transient ischemic attack, several weeks or even months before their strokes (most people don't know what a TIA is and therefore don't do anything to protect themselves).

AREAS TO TREAT/TYPES OF MANIPULATION

Work both feet completely first. Then find the locations of reflexes that correspond to these organs, and work in the following order (see Chapter 3 for guidance):

1. Head. Using the tip of the thumb, first work the tips of all the toes, using a circular motion; then work all around the whole toe. Concentrate on the tips (which correspond to the top of the head).
2. Spine: Holding the foot with one hand, glide the other thumb tip from the top to the bottom of the reflex.

These reflexology points can be used if you've had a stroke and are in the process of recovery or to prevent stroke if you've had a series of TIAs and may be at risk for stroke.

PREVENTIVE MEASURES AND COMPLEMENTARY TREATMENTS

Reflexology works well in conjunction with other alternative therapies and commonsense measures. For example:

GET REGULAR CHECKUPS: See a physician regularly for a blood pressure check and a baseline electrocardiogram (to test your heart function) at thirty-nine if you're a man and at fifty if you're a woman.

TAKE CARE OF CIRCULATORY PROBLEMS: If you do have high blood pressure or any circulatory problems, such as thrombophlebitis, take steps (diet, exercise, medication) to control them. Early detection of these problems can help protect you from stroke.

DO YOUR EXERCISES: If you've already had a stroke, speech and physical therapy is the way back to a normal life. You must first be able to overcome frustration and anger and to muster the commitment to relearn the most basic things. But the rewards, though slow in coming, will be worth all your effort.

If you experience periods of weakness down one side of your body or sudden loss of vision in one eye, see your physician at once.

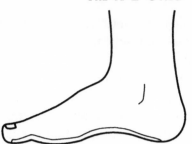

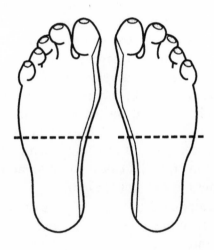

ULCER

Dinner was about an hour ago, and suddenly you've got this burning feeling right in the pit of your stomach. It can't be hunger pains—sometimes this lousy feeling wakes you up at night—and only an antacid or a cracker will alleviate the pain.

An ulcer is an open sore on the surface of the stomach, the esophagus, or, most commonly, the duodenum. Duodenal ulcers usually develop when an abundance of stomach acid and pepsin (an enzyme that breaks down protein) eats away at the tissue. This overproduction of acid may be triggered by smoking, ingesting too much alcohol, or repeatedly taking certain medications (aspirin being a chief culprit). Although stress will not in and of itself create an ulcer, it can add to the hostile environment that allows an ulcer to develop. Ulcers also tend to be hereditary; you may have a predisposition to developing one if a parent or grandparent had one.

Ulcers can also develop in the stomach (a gastric ulcer) because of an inherent weakness in the stomach wall. The alkaline mucus that is supposed to be produced by the lining of the stomach isn't sufficient to combat the amount of acid present. The same environmental factors that cause a duodenal ulcer may cause a weakness in the stomach wall.

Doctors used to keep patients on a completely bland diet, permitting no spices or foods that might irritate the gastrointestinal tract. The thinking these days, however, is that you may eat anything and everything that doesn't start up any symptoms.

SYMPTOMS: A burning sensation in the lower stomach about half an hour to several hours after eating or in the middle of the night, when stomach acids have built up sufficiently to irritate the nerve endings in the exposed sore. Other possible symptoms include pain in the chest or back, heartburn, nausea, vomiting, or constipation. A bleeding ulcer may cause blood in the vomit or the stools, weakness, or great thirst.

AREAS TO TREAT/TYPES OF MANIPULATION

Work both feet completely first. Then find the locations of reflexes that correspond to these organs, and work in the following order (see Chapter 3 for guidance):

1. Stomach: Apply gradual circular pressure with thumb tip and pad.
2. Solar Plexus/Diaphragm: With thumb tip, apply gradual pressure in the center of the reflex, and work out to the edges
3. Adrenals: Apply direct pressure with thumb tip.

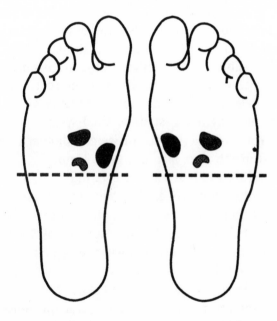

PREVENTIVE MEASURES AND COMPLEMENTARY TREATMENTS

Reflexology works well in conjunction with other alternative therapies and commonsense measures. For example:

DON'T EAT ANYTHING THAT UPSETS YOUR STOMACH: Although doctors these days don't restrict ulcer patients to "white" diets (cottage cheese, potatoes, and buttermilk—no spices), it's wise to listen to your body. If Mexican or Chinese food gives you a pain in your gut, by all means, don't touch it.

CUT OUT CAFFEINE AND NICOTINE: Both caffeine and cigarettes will irritate the lining of your intestinal tract and conceivably create more stomach acid, so eliminate both from your life and see if it makes a difference.

CALM DOWN: A program of meditation, visualization, yoga, or tai chi chuan will help you manage stress better. All the cells in your body, including those in your duodenum and stomach lining, function more effectively when the mind is calmer. Also, the enteric nervous system, a secondary system found in the stomach, is the one responsible for butterflies in the stomach and that knot we get when we're anxious. A more relaxed attitude can release a great deal of the tension we generally hold throughout our gastrointestinal system.

COAT YOUR STOMACH: Pepto-Bismol will coat the lining of the stomach and also contains bismuth, a metallic compound that kills some bacteria that may irritate the lining of the stomach and duodenum. (Some doctors think that these bacteria, rather than stomach acid, are the culprits that cause ulcers.) Pepto-Bismol is a short-term solution; your physician will prescribe medications that also coat the stomach.

Most ulcers can be managed with reflexology and other commonsense treatment most of the time. However, if you become severely nauseated and vomit blood or there are dark, grainy particles in the vomit, or if you pass black stools or stools tinged with blood, these may be signs of an ulcer that's bleeding internally. See your doctor immediately.

URINARY TRACT INFECTIONS (CYSTITIS)

You have to urinate, but you don't want to. As soon as you start, you know you'll be in agony. You always have to get up at night, and your lower back has been really sore lately.

Urinary tract infections (cystitis) are caused by bacteria that enter the urethra and pass into the bladder. Women are much more susceptible to this type of infection than men for several reasons. First, the bacteria have a very short distance to travel (about an inch and a half in women, as opposed to eight inches in men). Second, the openings to the vagina and anus are quite close, which means that bacteria can easily be transferred from one area to another, during either toileting or sex.

Another cause of cystitis, which may affect both sexes, is an obstruction in the urethra, caused by a kidney stone, a tumor, or (in men) an enlarged prostate gland. When a mineral deposit or growth blocks the passageway, the bladder can't empty properly, and the urine trapped there becomes a breeding ground for bacteria.

Finally, the urethral lining may have a weakness in it that allows bacteria to enter the urinary tract. Aggressive penetration during intercourse may damage the urethra, making it more likely to become a host for bacteria.

SYMPTOMS: Burning pain on urination, cloudy urine, urge to urinate frequently, blood in the urine.

Areas to Treat/Types of Manipulation

Work both feet completely first. Then find the locations of reflexes that correspond to these organs, and work in the following order (see Chapter 3 for guidance):

1. Kidneys: Apply direct pressure with thumb tip.
2. Adrenals: Apply direct pressure with thumb tip.
3. Ureter: Glide tip of thumb down ureter, from kidney to bladder.
4. Bladder: Apply circular pressure with thumb pad.
5. Spleen: Apply gradual circular pressure with thumb tip and pad.
6. Lymph Glands: Work thumb tip and pad gently back and forth across area.

Preventive Measures and Complementary Treatments

Reflexology works well in conjunction with other alternative therapies and commonsense measures. For example:

FLUSH THE AREA: To get the bacteria out of the bladder (and out of the urethra), you need to produce a lot of urine to keep flushing it out. (By not urinating often, you set up a breeding ground for *E. coli,* which doubles its population every twenty minutes.) So the more you drink, the more you go to the bathroom, the more bacteria get washed out—and the better you feel.

CONCENTRATE ON CRANBERRIES: Cranberry and cherry juice contain quinolinic acid, which converts to hippuric acid in the liver. This type of acid as well as the vitamin C in the juices has a positive impact on clearing up the infection.

URINATE BEFORE AND AFTER SEX: In the interests of removing any existing bacteria, go to the bathroom before intercourse. In the interest of flushing away any bacteria

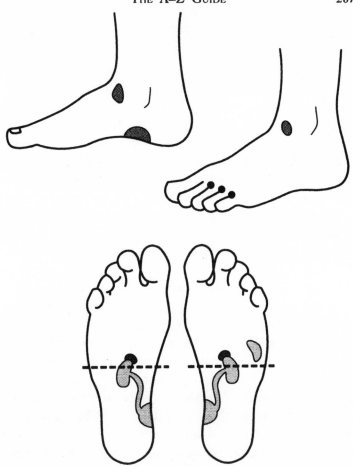

your partner's penis may push backward toward the bladder, go to the bathroom after sex.

WIPE CAREFULLY: Always remember to wipe yourself from front to back after defecating, so as not to spread bacteria from the anus forward to the vagina or urethra.

If the pain, burning, and blood in the urine have not responded to reflexology and other commonsense treatments, or if you have fever and nausea or vomiting, consult your physician, who may prescribe a course of antibiotics.

Varicose Veins

They look so ugly, like a road map scrawled down your legs. Those blue, swollen tracks are embarrassing, especially in the summer, when you're in shorts and bathing suits. Those little "spider" veins, the small red ones, are nearly as bad. Your legs feel almost as awful as they look; they ache whether you stand up or sit down.

Varicose veins aren't just a cosmetic problem; they are an indication that you have a circulation disorder. The blood supply pools in the legs, and this distorts the thin vein walls wherever there is pressure or weakness.

When your circulation is moving normally, the muscles act as a pump to return nonoxygenated blood from the legs to the heart. As the muscles contract, they squeeze the blood upward through a series of valves that work in only one direction. But if you've been standing for hours, and the muscles aren't contracting, the heart has to work very hard to pump blood upward against gravity. If the valves don't work properly, some blood travels back downward and stagnates in the veins, stretching them to the surface of the skin.

Varicose veins seem to run in families, and people with deep vein thrombosis may be predisposed to develop varicose veins as well (see Phlebitis, p. 234). Additional causes are standing on your feet all day, sitting with legs crossed all day, lack of exercise, obesity, and pregnancy. Women tend to be more susceptible than men, and this problem is even more common in tall women—since it takes the blood longer to get back up those long legs.

SYMPTOMS: Blue, distended swollen veins in the legs

(varicose veins in the rectal area are hemorrhoids, see p. 174), feelings of heaviness and achiness in the legs, swollen ankles, pain shooting down the legs, leg cramps at night. You may also develop a type of eczema, or scaling skin, right over the varicose veins.

Areas to Treat/Types of Manipulation

Work both feet completely first. Then find the locations of reflexes that correspond to these organs, and work in the following order (see Chapter 3 for guidance):

1. Colon: Beginning on the right foot, apply direct pressure with your thumb tip to the ileocecal valve; then glide the thumb tip from this valve up the ascending colon, across the transverse colon, to the inside edge of the foot.

   Switch to the left foot. Glide the thumb tip left to right across the transverse colon, down the descending colon, and end with a slight hook upward at the sigmoid colon.

2. Endocrine System (Adrenals, Ovaries or Testes, Thyroid/Parathyroid, pituitary):

   Adrenals: Apply direct pressure with thumb tip.

   Ovaries or Testes: Apply gradual circular pressure with thumb tip and pad.

   Thyroid/Parathyroid: Work "necks" of toes with thumb tip.

   Pituitary: Apply direct pressure with thumb tip.

Preventive Measures and Complementary Treatments

Reflexology works well in conjunction with other alternative therapies and commonsense measures. For example:

PUT YOUR FEET UP: Whenever you can, elevate your

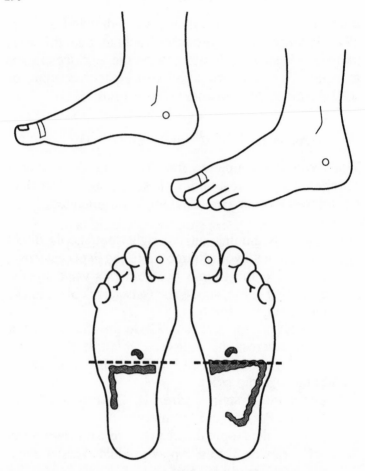

feet and legs above your hips. This way the blood will have an easier time finding its way back to your heart, and the heaviness and fatigue in your legs will dissipate.

WEAR ELASTIC: Support stockings can keep the blood from pooling in the small vessels close to the skin and bring it back to the deeper veins within the legs.

GET SOME EXERCISE: The more you move your legs, the better your circulation will be. If you've never exercised before, or if you're overweight and out of shape, start slowly with a daily walk—just as far as you can go without huffing and puffing. Every other day add another block. Other types of exercise, such as biking, swimming, or step training, will also make a difference to your legs.

CUT OUT CIGARETTES—AND BIRTH CONTROL PILLS: Smoking deprives the cells of oxygen and also may be a risk factor for the development of varicose veins. Birth control pills may create hormonal imbalances that in turn may help create spider veins.

Reflexology and commonsense measures may help alleviate the discomfort in your legs. However, if you have a severe case of varicose veins, you should consult your physician, who may recommend surgery (stripping the veins) or the injection of a chemical that closes off the distressed veins so that the blood can find other functioning venous avenues back to the heart.

VISION LOSS

You wipe your glasses, then blink, then wipe the glasses again. Everything's been looking blurry lately. It must be your mind playing tricks. It can't be possible—can it?—that you really can't see.

Vision loss is frightening, and there are a variety of problems that may cause it. As light enters the eye through the cornea, it curves the shaft, making it focus inward. The iris, which surrounds the pupil, then regulates the size of the pupil depending on the amount of light present, making the opening smaller if it's bright and larger if it's dark. The lens, which sits behind the iris, then fine-tunes the focus on the light and directs it to the light-sensitive rod and cone cells at the back of the eye. These cells change the incoming light to electrical impulses, which can be transmitted to the brain via the optic nerve.

If any of these structures is damaged or dysfunctional, the quality of vision changes. There are several different problems that may cause vision loss:

Amblyopia: This condition may occur in one or both eyes and refers to diminished vision, either from lazy eye, or strabismus, in which the eyes don't line up correctly, or from toxic amblyopia, which is generally a disease of chronic alcoholics (toxins from the alcohol irritate the optic nerve).

Astigmatism: When the shape of the lens is distorted, rays of light can't be properly focused on the retina, which makes the image go out of focus.

Cataract (see Cataracts, p. 89): This term refers to a clouding of the lens that results in loss of vision.

Detached Retina: If blood or other fluid from the eye collects between the retina and the choroid (the underlying layer of tissue that surrounds the retina), a hole may form in the retina, allowing the fluid to leak in. The retina will then detach itself from the choroid, causing dark spots, flashes, or streaks of light and eventual blurring of vision.

Glaucoma (see Glaucoma, p. 148): This condition is caused by increased pressure within the eyeball as the result of improper drainage of fluids. Vision loss is very gradual, usually proceeding slowly from the peripheral vision inward to the central vision.

Macular Degeneration: This condition results from the deterioration of the macula, the depression in the central part of the retina. Since the macula contains the most visual receptor cells of any part of the eye, its dysfunction almost always results in a loss of central vision (peripheral vision may stay intact, however).

Myopia (Nearsightedness): When the eyeball is too long, the cornea and lens focus the image in front of the retina, resulting in a fuzzy image.

Night Blindness: A vitamin A deficiency often causes the cones and rods in the back of the eye to lose the ability to distinguish fine detail and color of images as well as a sensitivity to adapt to loss of light on an object.

Retinopathy: This condition, which is common in diabetics and people with high blood pressure, involves a deterioration of the retina caused by retinal damage or overproduction of retinal blood vessels. It often triggers a hemorrhage in the eye, which may cause total blindness.

SYMPTOMS: Foggy or blurred vision (all conditions); visual disturbances, such as flashes and dark spots (detached retina); loss of central vision (cataract, glaucoma, macular degeneration); loss of peripheral vision (glaucoma); night blindness.

AREAS TO TREAT/TYPES OF MANIPULATION

Work both feet completely first. Then find the locations of reflexes that correspond to these organs, and work in the following order (see Chapter 3 for guidance):

1. Eye/Ear: Apply direct circular pressure with thumb tip.
2. Neck: Using thumb tip and index finger, manipulate "necks" of toes thoroughly.
3. Kidneys: Apply direct pressure with thumb tip.

PREVENTIVE MEASURES AND COMPLEMENTARY TREATMENTS

Reflexology works well in conjunction with other alternative therapies and commonsense measures. For example:

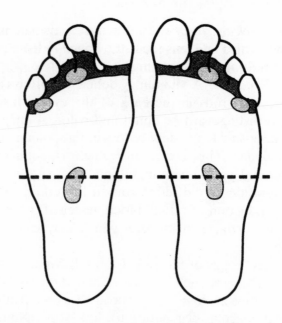

GET A CHECKUP: A yearly eye exam with a glaucoma screening is a wise preventive strategy for better vision. An optometrist, ophthalmologist, or optician can perform these simple tests and monitor the changes in your eyes over the years. This is particularly important for children and people in midlife (when the eyes may change considerably), but it's a good idea for everyone, no matter what age.

CONTROL YOUR BLOOD PRESSURE: Pressure throughout the body is the same inside the eyeball, and if yours is routinely higher than 140/90, you're potentially damaging the structures of your eye. A low-salt diet, daily exercise, and some form of stress management technique such as meditation or yoga can keep your pressure stable.

WEAR YOUR GLASSES: If you've been told that you're astigmatic or myopic and you need glasses, by all means wear them. Not doing so strains the eyes and may put you at risk for injuries or accidents.

MAKE LIFESTYLE CHANGES: Cigarettes and alcohol are toxic substances and in excess can damage many of the body's vital tissues. The eyes are particularly sensitive to chemical abuse, so cut down or cut out the substances that may damage your vision.

If reflexology and the alternative treatments mentioned above have not improved your vision, you should consult your physician for a diagnosis. Some conditions may need antibiotic treatment; others may require surgery.

WHIPLASH

You're just sitting in your car, minding your own business, when without any warning you are rammed from behind. The impact throws your body forward abruptly, but momentarily your head is left behind, then suddenly lurches forward to meet your body.

Whiplash is a sprain of the neck that occurs when the body is whipped violently from one position to another. It is almost always caused by a car accident, and it generally takes place when a vehicle at rest is hit from behind by a moving vehicle. The body in the front car is suddenly propelled forward, but the head doesn't catch up for a moment and bends backward. This can injure the muscles and ligaments of the neck and throat and tear small blood vessels in this area as well. (Whiplash injury can also occur during sports activities or any type of physical battering.)

In a bad accident you can dislocate one or more of the joints in the neck or even fracture neck bones. Most patients recover within a month. However, in severe cases pain and disability can last for a year or two. Many chiropractors and osteopaths think that once you have experienced this type of trauma to the neck, the cervical vertebrae may need ongoing adjustment so as not to create other problems farther down the spine. Many people have some arthritis in the neck joints that is triggered or exacerbated by such an accident.

SYMPTOMS: Immediately afterward you may have no symptoms at all, and pain may not start up until the day after the accident. At that point you might experience generalized neck pain that spreads to the shoulders or upper arms. It may feel difficult to move your neck up and down or around, and you may have muscle spasms.

In cases of severe injury accompanying symptoms, such as blurred vision, dizziness, headache, or difficulty in swallowing, may occur. These symptoms usually last only a few days. However, the pain, muscle spasms, and restricted movement can persist for months.

AREAS TO TREAT/TYPES OF MANIPULATION

Work both feet completely first. Then find the locations of reflexes that correspond to these organs, and work in the following order (see Chapter 3 for guidance):

1. Neck: Using thumb and index finger, manipulate "necks" of toes thoroughly.
2. Lungs: With the tip and edge of the thumb, work up and down and left to right.
3. Spine: Holding the foot with one hand, glide the other thumb tip from the top to the bottom of the reflex. Concentrate on the cervicals (the first third of your foot, from the big toe to just before the arch).

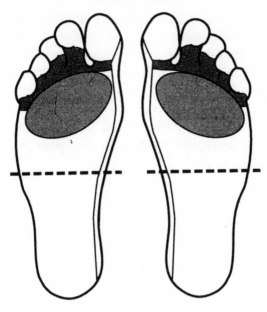

Preventive Measures and Complementary Treatments

Reflexology works well in conjunction with other alternative therapies and commonsense measures. For example:

ALWAYS WEAR A SEAT BELT: Don't drive around the corner without your belt attached. If you come to an abrupt stop, get into the habit of consciously trying to place your head against the headrest. That way, if you're rear-ended, you'll give your head and neck support automatically.

DO NECK ROLLS: Good preventive care for your neck means exercising it daily for flexibility and strength. First, drop your chin into your chest, and circle it to your right, trying to touch your ear to your shoulder. Reverse, circling left. Next, do diagonal stretches, aiming the top of your head to the upper right and your chin to the lower left. Reverse. Finally, put your chin straight down to your chest, lift to center, then place your head as far back as you can comfortably go, and come back to center.

WEAR A BRACE IF INJURED: A neck brace is insurance that you won't jerk your head involuntarily and worsen your injury. Wear it when you're awake, and your course of recovery will be faster.

If your pain is not alleviated by reflexology or the alternative therapies listed above, see your physician.

REFLEXOLOGY RESOURCES

REFLEXOLOGY NATIONAL ASSOCIATION

Reflexology Research Project
PO Box 35820, Station D
Albuquerque, NM 87176

This organization will give you information on where to study reflexology or find a reflexologist. It publishes a bimonthly newsletter called *Reflexology*. A subscription costs $12.50 a year.

HOLISTIC HEALTH ORGANIZATIONS

Center for Natural Medicine, Inc.
1330 SE 39th Ave.
Portland, OR 97214
(503) 232-1100

A consultation, research, and diagnostic center run by naturopathic physicians, offering a range of therapies

from naturopathy to chiropractic, acupuncture, homeopathic, and botanical medicine.

Rise Institute
PO Box 2733
Petaluma, CA 94973
(707) 765-2758

This educational organization offers courses, work-
shops, and seminars to help people cope with chronic
disease. The physical, emotional, and spiritual approach
of the healing is based on the work of Sri Eknath Eas-
waren, a meditation teacher who created his own program of natural healing.

American Holistic Health Association
PO Box 17400
Anaheim, CA 92817
(714) 779-6152

This organization publishes information on holistic
approaches to health care.

American Holistic Medical Association
4101 Lake Boone Trail, Suite 201
Raleigh, NC 27607
(919) 787-5146

This group of physicians dedicated to holistic medical
practices may offer referrals to doctors in your area who
are members.

Center for Mind-Body Studies
5225 Connecticut Ave. NW, Suite 414
Washington, DC 20015
(202) 966-7338

The center provides education and information for
anyone wishing to explore his or her capacity for self-

care and self-healing. It also sponsors self-help groups for people with chronic illnesses.

Mind-Body Medical Institute
Mercy Hospital and Medical Center
Stevenson Expressway at King Dr.
Chicago, IL 60616-2477
(312) 567-6700
This institute integrates Western medical practice with behavioral therapy in order to balance mind and body. An interdisciplinary staff works on wellness and illness care with patients.

Preventive Medicine Research Institute
900 Bridgeway, Suite 2
Sausalito, CA 94965
(415) 332-2525
This organization, founded by Dr. Dean Ornish, offers training programs and conducts research in mind-body medicine.

REFLEXOLOGY TOOLS

The Reflexology Decoder, Dynamo House Pty, Ltd.
  Australia
Available at the Natural Apothecary
105 Main St.
Brattleboro, VT 05301

Foot Roller Massager #624
NENS
New England Earthline Bodycare
Oceanside, NY 11572

Ma Roller
Awareness and Health
The Natural Apothecary
105 Main St.
Brattleboro, VT 05301

Foot Massager Roller
K-5048
Vermont Country Store
PO Box 128, Rte. 100
Weston, VT 05161

Ma Roller and Foot Massage Roller
Living Arts Catalog
PO Box 2939
Venice, CA 90291-2939
800-2-LIVING

Bibliography

Bayly, Doreen E., *Reflexology Today,* Thorsons Publishers, Rochester, VT, 1984.

Carter, Mildred, *Helping Yourself with Foot Reflexology,* Parker Publishing Co, Inc., West Nyack, NY, 1969.

Dougans, Inge, with Suzanne Ellis, *The Art of Reflexology,* Element Books, Rockport, ME, 1992.

Goosmann-Legger, Astrid I., *Zone Therapy Using Foot Massage,* Saffron Walder, The C. W. Daniel Company Ltd., Essex, England, 1986.

Kunz, Kevin, and Barbara Kunz, *Hand and Foot Reflexology: A Self-Help Guide,* Fireside/Simon & Schuster, New York, 1984, 1987, 1992.

Marquardt, Hanne, *Reflex Zone Therapy of the Feet: A Textbook for Therapists,* Thorsons Publishers Ltd., Rochester, VT, 1983.

Norman, Laura, with Thomas Cowan, *Feet First: A*

Guide to Foot Reflexology, Fireside/Simon & Schuster, New York, 1988.

Wills, Pauline, *The Reflexology Manual,* Healing Arts Press, Rochester, VT, 1995.

INDEX